Eating Problems: Alternative Solutions for Adults

by

Adey Mcsnotty

I0449578

ISBN: 978-1-326-65647-8

PublishNation
www.publishnation.co.uk

Contents

Introduction

How did it get to this? How did I let it get so far? I was driving to my local GP in tears. My wife had pretty much forced me to go. I tell you now, I rarely let my emotions get to me, and I seldom shed a tear. However, on the way to my appointment with my local GP, I was in floods of tears for a good fifteen minutes. I was a total mess.

I arrived and sat in the waiting room. I had been living with this condition for well over fifteen years but had never sought help from anyone. The first time that I had opened up to anyone about my situation was earlier in the day when I burst into tears in front of my wife at the dinner table. Explaining to my wife that I had been making myself sick for the last two weeks was certainly one of the most embarrassing moments of my life, if not *the* most embarrassing moment. I was utterly ashamed. The thing was that I had got to a point where I didn't know what to do. It was my worst nightmare, the only thing that I had ever had control of had finally started to beat me. I had puked up everything that I had eaten the previous day, and I didn't know how to stop. I couldn't keep this a secret any more. I had to tell my wife, the poor woman.

My name was called to see the doctor. This was the moment that I was absolutely dreading. Ironically, while I was waiting to be seen, I picked up a *Men's Health* magazine and saw an article that described the perfect diet. Surprisingly, this didn't make me feel any better whatsoever. I walked into the doctor's room and managed to just about keep it together. Then my bottom lip went and once again I burst into tears. On this day, I felt like a complete wet blanket. My emotions were everywhere. The doctor kindly pointed me in the direction of the tissues and, after what felt like forever, I explained to the doctor that I had been making myself sick.

Before making the appointment I thought that the doctor may not take me seriously, especially as I felt pretty fat. For that reason, I had asked my wife to gather a few photos together to show my drastic weight changes over the years. They were pictures that ranged from the age of ten into my early twenties. I also had a few more recent photos of me in my mid to late twenties, when I had gone through spells of quite drastic weight loss. The doctor was really kind and understanding. I told my wife before that I would refuse to see a male, as I was too embarrassed. However, my wife wanted to make me an emergency appointment and there were no female doctors available. I felt too ashamed to see a male. At the time, my sense of manhood was destroyed.

My reasons for writing this

So what is the reason behind writing this book? Well ... it's quite simple, really. There are two main reasons. The first reason is to raise as much awareness as possible about eating problems and disorders. If this book can support a person with an eating disorder in any way, or prevent a person from starting to have an eating problem, I will feel that it has all been worthwhile.

This may be a generalisation, but I feel that there is a stigma around eating problems. It's a grey area because there is no definite reason why they occur. And there is no medical cure. There are tablets and prescription drugs that can be used to help with the side effects and root problems, such as anxiety and depression. However, there is no definite answer. It can happen to anyone.

In terms of extremes it has become quite bad at times, but generally my eating problems are at the milder end of the spectrum. It has never got to the point where it has actually become life-threatening. I am certainly lucky in that way. The fact that I have managed to get into a good career (and keep myself busy) has certainly helped.

The second reason for writing this book is more personally therapeutic. A lot of the content in this book contains anecdotes and tales from my past, many of which I have kept to myself. I was always quite embarrassed by them, and failed to accept who I was. Being transparent and open will enable me to tell my story. By the end it will hopefully feel like a huge weight off my shoulders. As I said, I am not an extreme case. But I wouldn't want anyone else to suffer like I did at times.

While writing this book I decided to write very openly, on purpose. It's not an academic piece of writing that will be used for ground-breaking research. It's experience-led, which could support many people's knowledge of eating problems and disorders. This may include:

- People with eating problems
- Parents or carers of those with eating problems
- Friends of those with eating problems
- Professionals such as therapists, teachers, psychologists and doctors

- People with a general interest in learning about eating problems

Eating problems and disorders

I don't think there is any real need to differentiate between an eating problem and a disorder because they are basically the same. I believe that problems related to food make up part of a spectrum.

I currently work in education as a special educational needs and disabilities coordinator. As part of my role, I work with internal and external agencies to support lots of difficulties and disabilities including autism spectrum disorder, dyslexia, attention deficit disorder, dyspraxia and mental health. Where all the above come together is related to the fact that they affect people in varying degrees.

Let's take a difficulty related to food, which is what we are talking about. Imagine that you have an imaginary line from one to ten. You would classify number one as mild. Then you have number ten, which is severe. You could also have number five, which is moderate.

In order to get my views and opinions across clearly, I am going to use myself as an example. When I feel as if I have food under control there is still an underlying niggle, which constantly questions my food choices. This is something that I need to accept and to live with. So, with this in mind, I am still able to function in daily life. I can go to work, I can undertake daily chores, and I can socialise to varying degrees. So, because of this, I would be at the start of the scale, and the effects would be very mild.

Then, at the opposite end of the scale, imagine that you had severely reduced your food intake and that you were purging regularly. This way of life had become habitual, and the thoughts associated with this had become ingrained and extremely negative. All your family and friends were extremely concerned about both your appearance and your outlook on life. For this reason, a family member decided to seek medical help, as you had refused to admit your difficulties.

Although I have been going that way, my relationship with food has fortunately never become that serious, and I have never been hospitalised. So, with this analogy in mind, this extreme would be right at the top of the scale and it would be likely that these symptoms would be classified as a disorder. This is because the severity of need has a detrimental effect on your ability to function in daily life. You have basically lost control of your actions, and you need help quickly.

As I have implied, the severity of need related to food can certainly vary. However, it can very quickly spiral out of control. For example, someone may have started a diet with all the normal intentions to lose a few pounds. But then, very quickly, the control over their food intake has become addictive. However, this idea should not be generalised and can be dependent on your personality type. From my own experience, I have realised that eating problems are extremely complex, and it is very difficult to pinpoint the underlying cause. This is because the small amount of research undertaken has pointed to an array of factors. Factors such as self-esteem, anxiety, sexuality, genetics, and separation and loss are examples, but the list does certainly not end here.

So here it is: eating disorders are so complex that each case needs to be treated on its individual merit. I don't think that I would be alone in thinking this and this is not uncommon for other difficulties and disorders either. For example, each person on the autistic spectrum is completely individual. Yes, there are specific traits that are common, but that is about it. This is the same with eating problems and disorders.

Types of support and therapies

It is important to be true to yourself and to look inwards, especially when considering how you are going to support yourself with your eating problems. At the end of the day, only you can make the correct decision. Showing initiative will enable you to be in charge of making positive change. There are lots of ways of supporting recovery, whether it be from traditional methods, such as counselling – or more recent forms of therapy, such as cognitive behavioural therapy (CBT). In this book, I will focus on more alternative forms of therapy such as mindfulness-based approaches like meditation and hypnotherapy. However, I think that when you are considering seeking help, it is important to have a basic understanding of the main types of therapy that are available. For this reason, I am going to talk about each one in a little detail.

Counselling

Why do people go for counselling? There are many reasons why people may seek support through the means of counselling. At times it can be quite challenging to talk about eating problems and disorders with family members and people who are close to you. This is because the person is not neutral, and there is a strong chance that your family member or friend may not have the appropriate skill set or qualifications to support you. They may actually try to reassure you, but in most cases this is not what you actually need.

Counselling is based on the principle of empowerment. It aims to give you the fundamental skills to enable you to go about making positive change. It gives you responsibility, and gives you control over your future destiny. Along with this, counselling also tries to help and support people in selecting and identifying their own resources. For example, I am aware that one of my main attributes is my resilience – especially when things become quite difficult. This can be an extremely useful resource, especially when you need to focus on a problem such as an eating disorder to bring about change. On the other hand, it is important to be aware that this positive trait can actually turn into something counterproductive, such as stubbornness, if it is not supported carefully. And, to use another example, if you found yourself moving into an old habit such as binge eating, you may either move towards a resource such as resilience or towards stubbornness. This is where the skill of the counsellor comes into play, as they are able to empower the client.

The aim of any counsellor should be to help a client. He or she shouldn't play the role of a mentor or a coach, where there is an element of authority. The relationship should be seen as equal. In order to seek help, a client must have trust in the person that they are seeking help from. This is where I feel that it can be helpful to speak to someone in confidence.

What is counselling?

Counselling can mean different things to different people. However, there are underlying principles that most people can relate to. As I have mentioned before, counselling is confidential for both the facilitator and the client. It's unique, in the way that the relationship between the two people in the room is explicit. It should always be seen as non-judgemental. I suppose in some circumstances parents may be invited to attend sessions when the client is still classed as a minor. As I understand it, there are a few exceptions to the rule. There are also such things as counselling groups, who all have a similar desire or goal when it comes to empowerment and change. This approach may suit people who find one-to-one counselling a little intrusive, or even claustrophobic. Also, in the longer term, group counselling may be a stepping stone to moving towards one-to-one counselling.

It sounds quite impersonal, but the best way to describe counselling is that of a process. It involves active listening, which empowers clients to understand ways in which they can move their lives forward.

Finally, a counsellor needs to have the appropriate qualifications to be able to help people. Along with possessing the personality traits that would make the counsellor suited to the field, a counsellor must have the training to be able to support your area of development.

How does counselling differ from other helping activities? It is important to realise that counsellors shouldn't seek to offer advice. This is where helping differs from counselling. Counselling is a process of active listening that will lead to the client taking steps towards empowerment and will allow them to take control of helping themselves.

When a client chooses to seek advice from a counsellor there is always a reason for going: there is an expectation that something will come of it. However, there is no expectation in terms of the client's behaviour. There is no emotional gain for the client, and there should always be an objective. In comparison, a helper who is not trained may have a natural urge to judge or even offer advice. In some circumstances the advice might even be subjective, which is not at all helpful.

There is a clear difference between a counsellor and a helper. Whereas a helper may show sympathy and offer words of support, a counsellor will show empathy and will empower the client to make decisions.

Cognitive behavioural therapy

My knowledge of cognitive behavioural therapy is starting to develop, and I feel that this breakthrough therapy will hopefully allow complementary therapies such as hypnotherapy and meditation to be recognised and practised in mainstream health. CBT has undergone a huge amount of scientific research, and it is now common for GPs to make referrals for people with a wide range of problems including depression, anxiety and eating disorders, to name a few. From my perspective the aim of CBT is to alter the way that you think to bring about positive change. To enable yourself to do so, you must recognise the way that you think and what your patterns of behaviour are. Being aware of positive, negative and neutral thoughts enables you to make a choice about your behaviours. I believe that the use of questioning is powerful in CBT because, after experiencing questioning, you will realise in time that the thought processes which led to your behaviours can be easily changed. It seems to have had a positive result, and I will be interested to see how CBT can be combined effectively with meditation and hypnotherapy in the future.

Hypnotherapy

This is an area where I have been lucky enough to have undertaken quite a lot of professional training. Through various training providers, I have become deeply fascinated by the way that hypnotherapy can bring about positive change. The hypnotherapy courses were also always very practical, and they allowed me to experience hypnotherapy through the means of some amazing practitioners. Everyone has their own style, and this is something that I like so much about hypnotherapy. I am absolutely determined to resist the temptation to include evidence-based research, which is full of quotes. I have spent years doing this, and I have proved that I can write to the level required for a master's degree. I prefer to write from experience with regard to mindfulness because everyone's experience is always different. This is the beauty of life. However, it can make things a little complicated at times.

So what is hypnotherapy to me? I believe that it is a process of first calming the mind. This enables a practitioner to facilitate affirmation, which will ultimately result in positive change. It must, however, be stated that a client must have the desire and determination to bring about that change.

In my opinion, practising hypnotherapy is a skill and, when practised over and over again, it can be extremely effective. As I said, for a client to be receptive to hypnotherapy, they must be in a state to be able to do so. Their mind must have an open awareness where thought is controlled. A client also must have a certain amount of focus and attention. After all, they must be able to actively listen to the affirmations given by the therapist. As I said, a client must be in a calm frame of mind.

After having an initial consultation with the client, a hypnotherapist will gather some information, and will hopefully be able to gauge the approach they are going to take to ensure that the client is receptive. Ultimately, a hypnotherapist must decide what type of induction to use. Induction is a formal word used to describe the process of calming the client or gaining the client's attention and focus. This can be done in various ways and, understandably, it very much depends on the client's personality type. For example, one client may be quite anxious and would benefit from a longer induction which could include exercises that calm the breath. This may include counting exercises or simply being aware of the flow of the breath. In some cases, it is not uncommon to ask a client to take a number of deep inhalations and exhalations. This increases the circulation around the body, and it certainly can help. In a profound way it can help a client to gain some clarity. It can almost be motivation in the way that it suggests, "Come on. Let's take control of the situation and face this internally." A longer induction can normally last up to around twenty minutes or so.

Using the imagination can be very powerful in hypnotherapy, and this is why many people say that it can be very effective for both children and teenagers. This is because they have so much creativity and imagination. During inductions it is also common to use music in the background as this can be very relaxing indeed. A hypnotherapist may ask you what your favourite place is. Common answers are beaches, parks and woods. This information will be found out during an initial consultation. An experienced hypnotherapist will personalise a script which will help the client to engage with the process.

Along with longer and more calming inductions, there is sometimes a need to offer quicker inductions. This is especially useful for people who are quite restless and who struggle to sit for longer periods of time. Sometimes shorter inductions can be useful for people who see hypnotherapy as quite mystic and magical. The idea of a hypnotherapist being able to put them into trance in a few seconds can be quite appealing to some people. Of course, there is no real magic to hypnotherapy. It's about being able to facilitate positive affirmation. If a client wants to be hypnotised and they want to make change they will. The mind is extremely powerful, but hypnotherapy is an incredible skill that should be used only to help people.

To return to the shorter inductions, there are plenty of techniques which can include processes such as rapid eye movement and a fixed-eye induction. For example, during a fixed-eye induction there is normally a focus point on the wall. This could be anything that can keep your attention. By using specific language, and when the client focuses on the point for a period a time, they will notice that their eyes have started to go into overdrive and they will normally start to blink quite quickly. The hypnotherapist knows this and will ensure that the client is aware of this. Very quickly the eyes will start to tire, and it will be more comfortable to close them. There we go, it's as simple as that. The client is now ready to move on to receiving positive affirmation. It all sounds very simple, but in fact it takes a great deal of practice to really be confident in using the skills of hypnotherapy.

I would therefore certainly question how long it takes for hypnotherapy to work. I would also probably question the evidence of how using hypnotherapy as a complementary therapy can support you in certain areas, especially when it comes to eating problems and disorders. There is quite a lot of evidence to suggest that hypnotherapy can certainly support clients in breaking bad habits. This in particular seems to have had quite a lot of success. For example, a client may have a particular habit of eating a specific food such as chocolate, crisps or cheese. One of the keys is to find how the trigger occurs. In other words, you find out what exactly makes you eat the food. It may be a specific time of the day or it might be a feeling. The idea is to change the association or the feeling into something positive to the client. Once again, in very basic terms, instead of eating a chocolate at a specific time of the day, you may work with a client to associate this time of the day with eating a piece of fruit.

Some hypnotherapists use strategies that are similar to regression to support clients. Using timelines to find out where problems or habits first started can be used. However, I have never really found it beneficial and I find this approach a little dated. I know of quite a number of hypnotherapists who tend to stay away from this approach, as it can be both tiring for both the client and the therapist. For the client, it can bring up quite a lot of unnecessary memories. For the hypnotherapist … imagine using regression on twenty clients a week. It would be very draining.

Supporting someone with an eating problem or a disorder can be a very complicated process, and for that reason – unless the hypnotherapist has an extensive background of working with specific clients – this process alone is not sufficient to bring about long-term positive change. In my opinion, someone with an eating problem disorder may benefit from seeing a hypnotherapist to support them with common links such as anxiety or mild depression. Once again, I must stress that hypnotherapy should be used as well as other professional services, such as a GP or a nurse. As I mentioned, using calm inductions as well as positive affirmation can especially support people who are quite anxious.

Like everything in life, you have to work for it, and you have to want to make it happen. It simply won't come to you by doing nothing and sitting and waiting for it. This is exactly the same with hypnotherapy. In fact, I would be keen to challenge anyone who does suggest that all hypnotherapy isn't self-hypnosis. I believe that a hypnotherapist's job is to simply facilitate the process. This is because after one session of hypnotherapy you won't go away and simply expect everything to change. It just won't. If you were suffering from general anxiety you may have a session, and you may go away with some useful strategies. But you won't be instantly cured. You will need to work and implement those strategies on a daily basis. You may have been taught specific practices to prepare you for an event, or general practices to relieve stress and for you to be a little calmer. In fact, in relation to self-hypnosis, it is not too dissimilar to calming meditation. In this type of meditation it is initially goal-orientated as it aims to calm the mind. However, the important thing to be very aware of is that it will not permanently make you calmer if – say – you practised self-hypnosis over a two-week period. If you stopped practising, you would very quickly fall back into your old ways and habits after a while. As I said, you have to work for it.

Meditation

With my hand on my heart I can safely say that meditation is the best thing that has happened to me. It has transformed my life and the way that I approach everyday situations. I never realised it at the time but, unknowingly, I actually started to meditate at a very young age in my bedroom. Sometimes, when I felt I needed some time on my own, I would lie on my bed and stare at the ceiling. I really like silence and I feel very comfortable with it, even when I am in the company of close friends. When I was growing up I suppose that I used to become very nervous leading up to events such as tests, football matches or even speaking in front of people. Some people would assume that I was just really relaxed and chilled, but deep down I was very shy and not really sure of myself.

So what led me to walk into a Buddhist centre at the age of twenty-seven? Well, I suppose that you get to a point where you realise that you need to face yourself. Surely there would be something that could possibly lead to a calmer and more carefree life, wouldn't there? Actually it was the lead-up to my wedding. Although it was undoubtedly the best day and weekend celebration of my life, I was certainly out of my comfort zone. I mean, I generally dislike being the centre of attention and I wasn't particularly looking forward to giving a speech to 150 people in French. Also, any sense of anxiety or nervousness would always lead to an embarrassingly sweaty forehead. This sweaty forehead has been the bane of my life, and something that has actually prevented me from attending many social events. My close friends knew about it and would make a joke of it, which was fine. However, when I was with people who didn't know me too well I would actually feel as if the whole world was watching me. As I will mention throughout the four-week meditation challenge, the toilet was always my escape when going to restaurants, pubs and nightclubs.

Over the last four and a half years I have completed many courses in meditation. I have mainly learnt meditation techniques through various schools of Buddhism, but I have also learnt techniques and skills in more therapeutic settings. Many of the meditation techniques and breathing exercises stem from eastern meditative practices, but it's not just through Buddhism. Meditation was practised well before the time of Buddha's teachings.

I don't think I can do the art of meditation justice in this short section. Words can't describe it, as you just have to experience it for yourself. I have to say that over the years I have certainly built up a habit of trying new sports or hobbies and quickly moving on, but with meditation it has been different. It simply doesn't seem to go away. It's transformational.

I think that people mainly meditate for two reasons. One reason is to calm the mind and the other is to gain a greater insight into the nature of how things really are. Some would argue that you have to gain a certain amount of calmness before you can gain insight. It could be described as gradual. On the other hand, some would say that practising insight meditation alone is enough. At the end of the day, you must decide how you practise meditation.

Dieting

I need to be extremely direct here as I truly believe that dieting does not work. I say this purely through personal experience. I am appalled at how the media promote dieting, and how it still appears to be the most popular way of losing weight. Yes, there is evidence to suggest that in the short term you may be able to lose a large amount of weight. And guess what? Well, the likelihood is that you will put the weight back on just as quickly as you lost it. The media play a huge part in promoting stories of where people have lost huge amounts of weight, and they are applauded for their efforts. Understandably, young people pick up on this and want to be just like the celebrities. However, the problem is that a lot of dieting successes are exaggerated by the media in an attempt to sell their product. This is why blame shouldn't be directly placed on celebrities. After all, they have a right to live their lives as they please. However, people who have low self-esteem and aspiration look for success through dieting as this is the only thing that they feel they are good at. For me that was certainly the case. I didn't know anyone else who could diet as well as me. If I saw or met someone of a similar age who was slimmer than me I wanted to beat them, and I wanted to know their secret.

I had always been into music, and at seventeen I joined my first proper band. It was a rock 'n' roll band. There was a mini rock revolution in the late 1990s and the early 2000s, and we were keen to tap into that scene. The fashion at the time was to wear skinny jeans and extremely tight jeans. I remember making treks from Stoke to Manchester to buy my T-shirts. At the time they were the tightest and what I considered to be the coolest. Unlike nowadays, when you can find tight jeans in most fashionable clothes outlets, this wasn't really the case during my teen years. Therefore – you guessed it – I had to wear girls' jeans and T-shirts. As an alternative, to ensure that they were supertight, I would sometimes wear children's T-shirts. While writing this I am certainly thinking how bizarre I was but, unfortunately, my desire to be skinny had become out of control. I would never blame anyone directly for my eating problems, but certainly didn't feel that the music magazines that I read helped. Many of the people on the front covers were very slim, and I was unaware of the fact that all the photos were computer-generated images and had been edited. I also wasn't truly aware of the extent to which these people were taking illegal drugs. I didn't take drugs and, fortunately, never went down that road. However, some people may be inclined to if it would result in losing a large amount of weight.

In my opinion, dieting leads to binge eating. I remember over a period of time, especially in my teens and early twenties, when I literally refused to eat any chocolate or crisps. At one point, even if a little bit of chocolate or any crisps touched my lips by chance, I would feel that I had failed. This is mainly because of when I was younger I was very overweight and I would binge-eat, especially on crisps.

Obviously your everyday person who doesn't have a history of eating problems may see dieting as absolutely fine. However, everyone has cravings, no matter how small they are. I am not exactly sure why, to be honest with you. Maybe it is because when we were children we often associated foods like chocolate and crisps as rewards and, because of this, we would start to crave them. This is maybe something that needs to be considered – especially when thinking about one of the major themes of this book, which is moderation.

If you don't label food as good or bad, and there is no particular association between food and reward, then surely this could lessen cravings and desires. Many people have foods that they like and dislike, and people also associate foods with particular times of the day. Maybe it would be a little extreme to abolish all traditions of breakfast foods and foods that people associate with lunch and dinner. However, I have found that by almost contemplating an element of feeling away from food you can reduce your emotional attachment to it. For example, I have always felt very proud that people have always perceived me as being extremely healthy. However, this is certainly not true. In the past I have gone through periods of very rigid dieting and eating. Naturally, the body is constantly craving what it can't have, and you almost continue to punish yourself because you know that if you give in there will be no stopping you. Every so often I would fail, and I would give in to my desires. This may have been because I had a brainwave and temporarily realised that this approach was completely irrational and ludicrous. Or it may have been on an occasion when I felt a little faint. When I gave in and felt a major urge to indulge I knew that I only had a short period of time, and I would often eat in secret as I knew that I needed to make the most of such a short time window. After all, eating lots of snacks and treats over a short period of time in public would probably shock people. This would either be because they would be shocked by the amount of food and the speed at which I was eating it, or because they had perceived me as being an extremely healthy person.

So, once you have the desire to binge, what you start to eat isn't particularly important. It's the amount that you can actually get away with. Yes, it is likely that you binge on items of food that you particularly miss. Once you start you begin to not be really aware of your inhibitions. They almost start to become out of control, and the food takes over. You almost know that what is happening is not right – and maybe, on a couple of occasions, you will tell yourself that you want to stop – but these good intentions are very likely to give way to the desire to carry on eating.

I vividly remember a time when I was travelling in Australia. It was at Ayers Rock, and I had paid for a ten-day safari with a group of friends. It sounded absolutely great, but the thoughts of

"What am I going to eat?" and "Are people going to judge my eating habits?" always crossed my mind. During that period, I would only eat toast for breakfast: there wasn't much movement on that at all in my mind. The only other type of food that I might eat would be cereal. I didn't know this in advance but toast or cereal weren't available and were not part of the package. There were not many shops around and I had little money as I was on a strict budget. So, because of this, I made the decision to skip breakfast. I stayed in bed on purpose and explained to the people on the safari that I liked to sleep a lot. So my first meal of the day would be at around 1 p.m. and, to keep in line with my two meals a day, this would be the first time that I would eat. You would have thought that I might have made an exception because I was participating in something that was out of my routine. Unfortunately, I was in a particular period where this wasn't really possible for me mentally.

Lunchtime was communal meaning that we would mostly eat together. It's very easy to find a comfortable routine, and this is what had happened to me. I had to have two meals a day, and one of them had to be toast with plenty of butter. So, during the communal meals at 1 p.m., while everyone was eating full meals, I would look very strange when I just woke up and ate two pieces of bread. People who I didn't know would question my habits, and I would often make excuses such as "I'm not hungry," and "I'm not a massive fan of the food that is on offer."

It is extremely tiring, and to almost live a double life consumes your mind. You almost feel trapped, but at the same time you feel that you are winning. It's almost like a little competition. On the other hand, though, you can feel isolated and quite different from the crowd.

I will now return to the original point that I was trying to make: binge eating simply doesn't work. Like most desires the habit will get stronger, and there will eventually be a moment when your dieting gets out of control. In my opinion, and especially when you have problems in relation to food, you need to take a step back. A lot of the time people tend to label food as good or bad, and this certainly occurs from a very young age. There are probably foods that you absolutely love and there are types of food that you tend to stay away from – and that you certainly would stay away from at a pub or a restaurant. And there are also foods that you either like or dislike.

So the key is not to label food in this way, and just to see food as food. It's a way of functioning, and it gives you the energy to spend quality time with your family and friends. It also gives you the energy to take part in creative activities such as music, art, and sport etc. But food needn't be at the centre of everything that you do. When you diet, food is sometimes seen as a treat, especially as you tend to eat at certain times and you try to make the very most of what you eat. Therefore, you would rely on meals that you really enjoy because sometimes it would be a while until you next ate.

My awareness of food is now completely open, and I will no longer rule any type of food out. Because I meditated and spent time reflecting on my actions, I no longer label foods as being good or bad. In a positive way, I see food as an opportunity to socialise and to have interesting conversations with people. As opposed to before, when I would be very particular about what I ate, I now tend to eat – within reason – what I am given. Living with an amazing cook who cooks good, fresh food and different meals every night certainly helps, and I am lucky to have this. However, there are certainly plenty of books out there and online classes where you can learn how to cook.

Being able to eat – and allowing myself to eat – three meals a day with fruit in between has allowed me to focus on much more important aspects of my life. It is certainly very much a foundation of my day, but it's not something that constantly passes across my mind. I am able to focus on other areas of my life much more freely. Yes, there will be times when I have a dip – but no one is perfect. We all have good and bad days. But if I eat a piece of chocolate on a gloomy Monday, it doesn't mean that the rest of the day will be dedicated to eating awful food. No, because I now know that it is perfectly reasonable to have a little piece of chocolate every day or even every other day. In fact, by having this approach, I have lost weight without even trying, and I actually feel healthier.

Vegetarianism

I generally believe that there are two reasons why people choose to become a vegetarian. The first reason is because people feel that by being a vegetarian they have more chance of losing weight. The second reason for becoming a vegetarian is for ethical reasons: people feel that eating meat is cruel and not particularly beneficial for the environment.

Now I have personal experience of both. Between the ages of twelve and twenty-three, my main reason for being a vegetarian was to lose weight. I felt that eating less protein would prevent me from putting on weight. On the other hand, between the ages of twenty-six and thirty-one, my reason for being a vegetarian was more to do with ethical reasons (along with my social circle).

For half my life I have absolutely dedicated myself to vegetarianism, and I have no regrets about this at all. If I was an outstanding cook and I had plenty of time on my hands … then yes, I would be a vegetarian – and probably even a vegan. However, I have realised that I am simply not skilled enough to feed myself the right nutrients because of my lifestyle. Also, for family and social reasons, I feel that I need to eat meat for my general well-being.

I will first discuss becoming a vegetarian for the reason of losing weight. In effect you have started a diet as soon as you decide to become a vegetarian because you are narrowing your options in terms of food choice. And because your reason for not eating meat is to lose weight, then there is every chance that over time you could start to cut out food groups such as carbohydrates. As I am sure you are aware, this is one of the necessary food groups, and consuming bread or potatoes goes to make a well-nourished individual. If you do not eat starchy foods your food choices can start to diminish very easily, which can lead to a low calorie intake. Also, because your food choices are reduced, you may start to eat foods that you can rely on. Some people would class these as comfort foods.

My experience of this was very similar and, because I became extremely picky with food choices, my options were extremely reduced. I very quickly defeated all the very well-researched benefits of being a vegetarian, as I would tend to eat dishes such as pizza and pasta because they would fill me up. Some people may suggest that by reducing your food options and choice you can readily maintain a weight that you are comfortable with. For example, if you ate two pieces of toast, a banana and a whole cheese and tomato pizza every day, you would maintain the same weight (you would have to take into account how active your life was on a daily basis as well, though). However, if you dieted like this you would crash and burn in the long term, especially when your food choices went out of your control. And this ideology is simply not healthy as you would definitely be missing out on a lot of vital nutrients.

Secondly, I will now start to discuss why people choose to become a vegetarian for ethical reasons. For me, it was when I started to become interested in meditation. In my experience, the more time that you spend meditating the more you start to consider your value as a person, as well as the value of other people. And at that time I was meditating with dedicated Buddhists and monks, so I was receptive to their thoughts and points of view. It's like peeling an orange. When you start to meditate you have many different layers and your thoughts are generally clouded and distorted. As time goes on you meditate more. As this happens the peel around the orange is peeled away, and you start to get somewhere near the bare bones of your true nature. It generally makes you question ethical principles, and this is particularly true when it come to your food choices.

You become more compassionate towards yourself and towards others when you meditate, and this includes all living creatures. Naturally, after a while, one would question the ethical reasoning behind eating meat. This is what happened to me. I generally enjoyed eating meat but I made the conscious decision to stop doing so. This was because in my state of awareness at that time, I felt that it was the most ethical decision to make. However, like everything, you often question your decisions, and this was certainly the case with vegetarianism. With most ventures I am always 100 per cent dedicated and don't commit to things by half. I am certainly an all-or-nothing type of guy.

Between the ages of twenty-six and thirty-one, I pretty much meditated every day and followed many of the precepts of a Buddhist monk.

However, I had a couple of children during that period so there were certainly some exceptions to the rules.

To return to vegetarianism ... there are definitely some stumbling blocks, and especially when it comes to social events. For example, my wife's friend invites us for a meal on a Sunday afternoon. In the UK we traditionally eat a Sunday roast which normally consists of a large piece of meat. Now here is the dilemma. You currently do not eat meat, but is there an argument to make an exception? Well, I suppose after being invited to a meal you could inform your wife's friend that you do not eat meat and you would like to request an alternative. Now some people might embrace difference and they might have a sound knowledge of vegetarian food, but for others this might not be the case at all. I have known some people become quite anxious leading up to the event and spend hours on the Internet while wondering what to cook for their vegetarian guest. This is not healthy, and, with regard to kindness and compassion to the host, you should question your decision to request an alternative.

Over time I have certainly altered my view of this type of situation. I simply accept the food that has been given to me. I think of it, in a way, like an alms bowl. Yes, if I have the choice, I am more than likely to go for a vegetarian option … but if someone has invited me for a meal which has taken hours to prepare then I feel that on these occasions it is more ethical to eat what is given to you. This is especially the case when you know the cook has a limited knowledge of vegetarian cuisine.

Retreats

You can go on many types of retreat. I suppose that the central theme of all retreats is to provide help for you. Here are two particular types of retreat that you can undertake: these are group retreats or solitary retreats. Each is an amazing but completely different experience in itself.

I will firstly talk about a group retreat. The number of people who attend will depend on many factors, such as the time of year and the main theme. I have been on retreats where there have been as many as sixty people and as few as ten. Sometimes it might be an idea to attend with a friend, especially if you are feeling a little apprehensive and you really don't know what to expect. On the other hand, though, every single person on the retreat who is attending for the first time probably feels exactly the same as you.

When you arrive at your retreat destination, you often have a little time to settle before meeting as a whole group to discuss the theme and the aim of a retreat. By the way, the reason why I am trying to give quite a lot of detail is because I actually felt pretty nervous before attending my first retreat. I certainly didn't know what to expect, and on the second day of a week-long retreat I decided to go home because it felt quite overwhelming. However, I quickly picked myself up and managed to jump back on board.

Let's get back to a group retreat. Sleeping arrangements play a big role in the success of a retreat. It is very normal to share a room with other people, normally up to around four others. This was the case on my first retreat. We slept in bunk beds. When I visited a Zen monastery we slept in the meditation hall where there were around thirty other people. Females and males were separated by a large curtain. However, here is something to be very aware of. There is a strong possibility that there will be a phantom snorer. And when I say a snorer I mean an almighty snorer. Now if you have been put in a meditation hall it is slightly more difficult to put a request in to change rooms, but if you are sharing with four other people this is certainly possible. You may feel as if you are being a little fussy, but you certainly shouldn't feel like this. Although you need to think of others and to feel a sense of compassion, it is likely that you don't have that many opportunities to participate in such an experience, and you won't want it ruined by a bad night's sleep. Therefore, it is important to speak up and request either an alternative room on your own or with another group.

To resolve any uncertainties you may have, you are normally given a schedule of the daily activities during the introductory meeting. This will almost certainly include activities such as sitting meditation, talks, group workshops, working/walking meditation and free time for reflection. This list is not exhaustive and there are certainly other activities that take place.

People often associate the term 'retreat' with hiding yourself away in a hut or going to the Himalayas for an extended period of time. This can be the case, and some experienced meditators may choose to go on retreat in the conditions above. But for many of us this is simply not possible. People have commitments such as family, work and friends. However, if there is ever an opening, or you have an opportunity, I would highly recommend going on a retreat.

What is a retreat and how would I define it? Well, I suppose I would say that it is taking a break for a period of time which is out of your normal, everyday routine. By doing so it gives you an opportunity to rest the mind, which will enable you to reflect on certain aspects of your life. Ultimately, this will allow you to jump back into your hectic life with a new sense of perspective and energy.

I am talking about this idea of taking a break from your normal routine, but for a retreat to have any long-term impact you must create certain conditions. Firstly, you need to remove every stimulus to give your mind, your consciousness and your thoughts a break. I would strongly recommend refraining from using electronic gadgets and software. And, yes, this does include mobile phones and television. I would also encourage you to even cut out things like music too. Now this might seem like someone's worst nightmare and you may find it extremely difficult. Refraining from using mobile phones will be likely to prove challenging because of the environment we live in. However, with a little bit of persistence, it can prove to be extremely rewarding.

The longest period of time I have spent on retreats is five days. Because of my lifestyle, this is really the maximum length of time that I could ever commit to. For me the first day was always very difficult, and this is because of the transition of going from a very hectic lifestyle to almost complete tranquillity. I had to remind myself that my mind was in absolute overdrive and that on the retreat time was no longer distorted, and the time went very slowly indeed. There were so many occasions when I wanted to grab my mobile phone or I would question myself and ask, "What am I doing here? Is it actually worth it?" With persistence and self-encouragement, you tell yourself that going on retreat is certainly a worthwhile activity to pursue and to take part in.

Going on retreat is unique, especially the dedicated period of time when you have absolutely no commitments at all. You have dedicated a set period of time to yourself and your self-development. Often people go on holiday and, for example, you may go on an all-inclusive holiday. However, when you return you certainly don't feel energised or relaxed. Yes, you have experienced a change of scenery, and you may have spent time with people who you dearly care about, but you have probably still experienced the stress of travelling, of packing your suitcase and of many other factors. Also, your food intake may have been excessive and you may have overused your mobile phone and watched too much television. Therefore, in my opinion, going on holiday may give your mind a break but it will never give you any real insight into moving forward with the stumbling blocks in your life.

From my experience, going on a solitary retreat is a completely different experience in comparison to going on a group retreat. For obvious reasons, for the time that you are on a solitary retreat you should have no communication with anybody. It is not uncommon for this to occur on a group retreat that is longer than a day or a weekend. Normally, after people have settled into their accommodation and have had time to have an introductory chat, the people on group retreats often simmer down into minimal conversation and sometimes silence. From my direct experience, it has been incredible to realise that after being on a short group retreat, without even talking to many people, I had connected with them in some way. It's really difficult to put this into words, though, and I suppose you would need to experience it for yourself to have an understanding of what I am referring to.

Unlike group retreats, during a solitary retreat you are solely responsible for your schedule. Absolutely no one will be watching you, so you will need to take full responsibility for all your actions. Of course it can be extremely easy to go off-task and undertake actions that don't really help or support the purpose of the retreat. At the start of the retreat, and during the evening, there might be an extremely strong desire to indulge. This may be because you are extremely bored, or it might be because you have very poor willpower at the time. Resilience is extremely important, and the power of this mustn't be underestimated.

Instead of going into a retreat somewhat blind, I would strongly recommend creating a short schedule, and I would be tempted to be quite rigid with this. Having minimal negotiation will reduce the temptation to go off-track. You have to be aware that you are more than likely to be in charge of your own food intake. Therefore, it is extremely important that you are well-organised. When it comes to writing your schedule, I would advise writing down exactly what you are going to eat and what time you are going to do so. By doing this it will ensure that food doesn't take over the retreat and fully occupy your mind. Where possible you need to minimise any anxiety related to this.

When you are planning your solitary retreat, I would always recommend letting people having an emergency contact number so that people can get in touch with you if needed. For this reason, you should take your phone. But, as I have already mentioned, you must have resilience and not give in to the temptation to take a quick look at it.

To summarise: given the chance (and depending on your lifestyle), I would strongly recommend going on retreat now and again. It re-energises you and it gives you the chance to recharge your batteries. Lengthier retreats also give you the opportunity to be in touch with yourself. It can almost take you back to the core principles and fundamentals of your being.

Exercise and running

I suppose that one of the main aims of exercise is to improve your social, physical and mental well-being. Overall I agree with this statement, but I think that the thought processes and ideas behind this often become somewhat confused.

I have run from an early age. If I remember correctly my original reason for starting to run was to lose weight. I think I was around twelve years old. I had always exercised and I played football to a good standard. When I first started to run I very much struggled and I couldn't keep going for ten minutes. It was quite embarrassing. However, in today's society this isn't uncommon, and because I am a qualified physical education teacher I have first-hand experience of this. It was saddening. During the last academic year we were lucky enough to be able to take our pupils to the beach to complete a short run that would take no longer than twelve minutes. With no exaggeration at all, over half of the pupils could not run or even jog continuously. They had to stop at least once. This was extremely saddening to see, and it made me consider where we were going wrong.

As I mentioned before, I used to run because I wanted to lose weight. It was directly linked to my problems and associations with food. Sometimes, when I had eaten a large meal, I would go for a long run to make sure that I would not put weight on. It's crazy, though, because straight after going for a run I would always weigh myself, thinking that I would lose weight or maintain my weight after going for a run. I now consider how I used to think and I can't actually believe how my brain used to work. It was a thought process that had somehow become automatic thinking. Also, this thought process would be exactly the same when I had been drinking alcohol the night before or if I wanted to treat myself with a chocolate bar – I would go for a huge run. I was absolutely terrified of gaining weight in my teenage years and early twenties.

My relationship with running has changed quite recently, and it has been transformational. I now actually enjoy going for a run. Who would have thought it? Very much like my relationship with most things, I was an all-or-nothing sort of guy. I would often run at a high intensity over a period of time, and would run at pace while timing my runs as well as measuring the distances. Needless to say, because of the increased intensity over a short period of time, I would burn out. I would have sore knees and my weak ankles would turn into glass. All in all, it wasn't a very nice experience. In essence, there was no element of moderation. My running was extremely goal-orientated, and I was really not showing any compassion to my social, physical and mental well-being.

You would think that as a qualified PE teacher I would relish competition – and I actually do, especially when it comes to sports such as football, tennis and badminton. My relationship with running is different as I often used it as a form of escapism. I would often listen to loud music and run through busy streets. By doing this I wasn't in touch with myself. By listening to loud music and running at a fast pace I had lost touch with my current state of consciousness. This would result in me returning home even more stressed and anxious than before.

So here it is: I am going to call it goalless running. The theory behind it is that there is no desired result. There is no aim, no training programme nor any weight target. Like a meditation technique such as just sitting or zazen, in this case the process is 'just running'. My experience of this has been immensely positive. It is the first time in my life that I have actually been able to say that I enjoy going for a jog. The amazing thing about 'just running' is that absolutely anyone can participate regardless of age or fitness levels. This is because the movement that takes place is no more than a light jog. You need to actually practise as if you were jogging but the speed is, debatably, no quicker than a very brisk walk. Even when I have jogged for over an hour I honestly feel invincible – so much so that I feel as if I could keep on jogging for hours.

Quite recently I read about an incredible Zen monk who sought enlightenment through something very similar to 'just running'. One of his jobs was to send post around the local area. It was a long round but he decided to extend it. For this reason, the crazy man decided to commit to running a marathon every day for a year. As I mentioned at the start, he set no real time limits. Although he had a goal, which was that he wanted to become enlightened (although arguably being enlightened is goalless), he wasn't participating for material gains. Deep down, he was simply looking for internal peace.

I normally jog for around an hour, but this really isn't of great importance. If I only ran for fifty-eight minutes then that would be OK. Maybe in the past I would have run for an extra two minutes just to prove to myself that I could do something. This is something that I found extremely interesting when visiting a Zen monastery. During the daily life of a Zen monk you participate in something called working meditation, and you set a certain amount of time per day to participate in it. However, when the planned amount of time has finished, you stop what you are doing, pack away and maybe prepare for another formal sit which involves staring at a wall in deep contemplation. Now the point is that even if you haven't finished, it doesn't matter. You simply let go. There is always another day. You haven't won or lost. You are where you are in the process of work.

An important aspect of goalless running is to leave space in between your allocated space and the amount of time that you have given to your practice. This is imperative because you certainly don't want to feel rushed. My life can be quite busy at times, what with bringing up a young family and having a professional management role in education. Sometimes I feel that time is not of the essence. In my current circumstances I make sure that my beautiful children are cosy and tucked up in bed which is normally at 7 p.m. I also try to organise times with my wife to ensure that we don't have any immediate plans for the evening. By doing this I can dedicate my space and compassion to mindful wisdom.

I remember a few years ago that I had signed up to go on a meditation retreat. It was a week long and at the time I didn't have children. However, I had a lot of schoolwork to do and I had been contemplating for nearly two weeks whether I should go or not. I arrived at the retreat and only lasted for two days. It was purely down to the fact that my thoughts were not correctly channelled. My thought processes had become fixated on the fact that I needed to get my work done. I knew that really it could have waited and, deep down, it was down to external factors as I wasn't ready to face up to things like my eating problems. However, that is something that you can find out more as you read on. The point I am reiterating is that your practice of goalless running must be respected, as you don't want to feel at all rushed.

I think it is essential to consider the time at which you prefer to run. And how often are you going to run? I know for a fact that I prefer to run in the evening. To keep the momentum going, I naturally started to jog every other day. I didn't particularly need a rest day but, for reasons of my own, this suited me best. Each person is truly individual and this is why you need to be true to yourself. I am lucky enough to have up to thirteen weeks holiday a year because I currently work as a teacher. For this reason I tend to be more proactive in terms of jogging during these times. Although it was for a particular reason, I generally do find this form of jogging extremely relaxing.

One of the main reasons behind this is because I am extremely aware of my surroundings when I jog. Every morning I drive along the same road as I make my way out of Norwich towards Great Yarmouth. I drive along this same street every single weekday, and I am extremely indifferent to my surroundings. Apart from the fact that I am half asleep (because it is very early in the morning) I travel by car, which means that I don't get to appreciate what is around me. This is a great shame because there is natural beauty in everything that we come into contact with. That's my opinion anyway.

When I undertake goalless running, because my attention is not focused on anything that has happened in the past – nor am I focused on anything in the present – I normally (after around half an hour) start to become aware of what is happening in that particular moment. Of course it wavers and nothing is ever constant, but there are glimpses. So, on my regular route, I tend to pass the area where I normally zoom past at those high speeds during those sleepy mornings. My experience is unimaginably different. This is because I am able to appreciate things and objects like the beautiful buildings, the natural wildlife, the changes in the weather and the delightful scenery in general. This really enables me to be aware of a person's own perception of the world. It can be completely different depending on your thoughts at the time. I can certainly relate to other aspects of my life too.

I am lucky enough to have my own office. It's on the second floor, and I have a direct view of the sea. At times it is absolutely beautiful, and on a summer's day it truly can be picturesque. People often come into my office and they are extremely envious of the fact that I have a beautiful view. Unfortunately, I often forget that I associate the office with work-related matters, and I spend a large amount of time either on the phone, on the computer or in meetings. This, once again, is my thought process and it's my perception. When people remind of the beauty of my sea view I try to take notice of this, and I try to think of ways in which I can be more in touch with how lucky I am.

I decided to try dedicating a certain amount of time per day just looking at the sea view, while having in mind that these mindful breaks will allow for more time to be productive. Regardless of how busy I was, I found that by taking time out, but only for a few minutes, gave my mind much more space to be creative. Because of this, the short breaks allowed for more productivity as my outlook was more positive. I think that I have made my point. Your outlook on your world is completely dependent upon how you perceive it.

I have – and will mention a number of times throughout this book – that when I can I enjoy contemplating, whether it's through the means of a formal meditation, a solitary walk, goalless running or even simply sitting with a cup of tea in my favourite chair, each experience is different, but they all aim to result in a calmer mind. When these practices are prolonged, depending on the conditions that exist, they may also result in insight. However, because I have a general preference for this type of approach, it doesn't mean that other concentration practices such as following the breath or affirming positive emotion are not as effective. They certainly have their place and I have spent a large amount of time practising them, both on my own and during longer and solitary retreats. Without trying to confuse you too much, I believe that an experienced meditator is able to combine all three approaches of breathing, positive emotion and contemplation into one practice.

When I go for a run, depending on my levels of concentration, I tend to practise all three types of meditation. When I leave my house I don't commit to one form of meditation to base my run on. It tends to be intuitive. When I say this I think that you shouldn't search for a meditation, but you should just let it come naturally to you. This was the same approach that I took during my four-week challenge. After I got out of bed early in the morning, I simply sat on my cushion and the meditation began. I think that it is important not to question things too much. Otherwise this can defeat the object of practices like meditation and even hypnotherapy. If you think too much it can result in thought reactions such as anxiety – which is quite contradictory, as this defeats the object of practising. Choice is a funny old conundrum and this is something that I will also mention in this book, especially when it comes to food and habits.

So, for practical reasons, I decided to go for a run that Monday evening. It had been a long old day and I didn't manage to have a lunch break as I had had a meeting that went on for longer than expected. Since I left the house that morning, it was literally the first time that I had spent any time on my own.

As I mentioned before, do not push or force an experience.

So I leave the house and I start to move. My pace literally feels as if it is everywhere. My mind is telling me to speed up as I want to go home and sit on the couch. All this is a complete illusion, and this is a mind-set that I need to manage. I don't necessarily feel that contemplation is the answer here. The mind needs to calm itself to allow the body to relax too.

In order to allow this to happen, a concentration exercise would be beneficial. You can vary your approach when following the breath, adding a count, following the length of the breath, or simply being aware of the cycle. It's up to you. Normally the time that it needs to be practised for will depend on the type of day that you have had. You may find that after ten minutes your mind starts to calm and you start to find a steady rhythm. To almost feel as if you are watching yourself run would be beneficial. I have sometimes had similar feelings when I undertake everyday activities which are automatic, such as washing dishes, riding a bike or sometimes even driving a car (a little scary). As I have mentioned, my journey to work currently takes around forty-five minutes, and because I have taken the same route every day for six years I sometimes lose track of my journey. Time is often distorted, as I often feel on autopilot. You are actually looking for something different, and although running will eventually feel like an automatic practice you will eventually be extremely aware of each moment. This takes some practice and quite a lot of sessions, though.

It is often extremely easy to give up and think to yourself that – really – this whole mindful approach and meditation is all a little bit airy-fairy. This is far from the truth, though. It is simply your mind almost playing with you, especially when things may seem a little tough. This will happen frequently at the beginning of the process. This is mainly because the concept of goalless running is almost alien to many of us. And in the face of potential failure many people will often consider giving up. Think about the idea of leaving the house and running regardless of whether it's raining, snowing, windy or blistering hot. Surely, it would be easier to simply sit in front of the fire watching an undemanding soap with a cup of your favourite drink, wouldn't it? Well, yes, in the short term, I believe that it may well be easier. But, in the longer term, if you choose not to consider alternative ways of calming the mind you may well face a lifetime of low-level to higher levels of suffering. This seems like quite a bold statement but it is simply true, and I can vouch for this through pure experience.

An hour of running may seem a bit too long, especially for those who seldom participate in exercise on a regular basis. You may want to gradually build it up. Over the course of a few weeks you could aim at completing twenty minutes, and then you could gradually build up to an hour. It is completely up to you because all elements of practice should be personalised and individual to each of us. However, in my opinion, I don't think that it is necessarily productive to gradually build up your practice. This is because, once again, it brings in an element of being goal-orientated. I mean that the pace at which you should run should be no more than an extremely light jog or just a little more than a brisk walk. And, for whatever reason, if you struggle with that, you can slow it down even further. Walk if you need to. After all, this should not be a painful practice. In fact it should be, and will eventually be, overall, a very enjoyable experience.

It is important not to be hard on yourself as I can guarantee that there will be setbacks. This is exactly the same as mindful eating. There will be times when everything goes out of the window. The important thing to do is to recognise that this is actually happening. Also, once in a while I would suggest that it could actually be a useful practice to do. For example, you have been extremely mindful with regard to your running and eating habits. Things seem to be going swimmingly well, and you feel as if you are making excellent progress, but at the back of your mind you almost feel a sense of mundane boredom. Well, why not indulge yourself? After all, the mind is training itself to have things that you can't have. I have done this before, particularly when I have felt a little isolated from the world. It's almost good to check in to see how the majority of people currently live in the Western world. This is not at all a criticism or a personal dig. It is simply the way things are.

Thoughts and mood can really have an effect on your experience of goalless running, but I must stress that it is important not to think that you are a superhero when you feel that you have experienced an amazing run. By all means experience the joy and certainly do not reject it. You must congratulate yourself when completing a successful run. Plus, on the other side of this, you must not beat yourself up too much if your run doesn't go to plan. For example, your experience may seem completely negative because a car carved you up when you tried to cross the road. The key is to focus, if possible, on moderating your whole experience. If you imagine water coming out of a tap at a steady pace (or even the cycle of the breath when it is calmed) you will see that it flows at a regular rate. When people fluctuate between highs and lows, I imagine that this could lead to eventual blowouts. If possible, it would be beneficial to treat each goalless run as just a run. That is all. You experienced your mind, your consciousness and your thoughts. That is it.

The four-week challenge

Week 1

Day 1

My alarm went off at exactly 5 a.m. You guessed it: my first thought was to place my head back onto my cosy pillow and have an extra hour and a half in bed. It was my first day back at work after a holiday, and who would really blame me if I had gone back to sleep?

I was thinking that if I was serious about making change, it needed to be radical. At this point my wife was in control of my food intake. I wasn't in a position at all to control it myself. What I was eating didn't particularly matter. This was by no means a long-term solution. This would not be fair on either me or my wife. For me, in a way, it would feel that I was a prisoner with regard to what I could eat. For my wife … well, I imagine that it would eventually become a bit of a burden. I needed to do this for myself, but before I could do so I needed support.

As my alarm went off there was a sense of urgency, a sense that I needed to get out of bed to help myself. The day before I had pledged to wake up at 5 a.m. every day to meditate and contemplate in order to aid my recovery from my latest setback. I would often suggest drastic changes – and my mind was everywhere at that moment, racing from one thought to another and thinking of as many things as possible to not face what was right in front of me: my eating disorder.

I crept downstairs, made a quick trip to the toilet, and put my phone on charge. I set up my meditation timer for forty minutes. I needed to start somewhere with my meditation because over the last three months it had been quite sporadic, with me meditating for twenty minutes here and there when I had a chance. Waking up at 5 a.m. was the perfect time to create the space and time to meditate. There was absolutely no rush, and it was completely silent. I had created the perfect conditions to support my change. Well … for today anyway. I was feeling quite self-centred, and every thought was currently about me and my problems, the fact that I had no control over my food and the facts that I both hated the way that I looked and I couldn't understand why I was not at the weight that I wanted to be.

So I knelt on my meditation stool, corrected my posture, got comfortable and closed my eyes. People often think that meditation is relaxing. This is true in many ways, but if you want to create real change you must pass through some pretty dark places to realise your true being. I just sat for the first ten minutes to prepare myself for the main part of the meditation. I suppose it was not too dissimilar to a body scan. I needed to arrive to enable my mind to be receptive to the practice that I was about to attempt.

I started with a loving kindness meditation. Because of the state I was in I had lost touch with humanity, and my love for myself and others needed to be found again. I needed to become less isolated from society, in a way, and I needed to connect with others. I had become obsessed with my ego. The loving kindness meditation that I am aware of involves naturally being aware of the breath while using positive affirmations to wish loving kindness to yourself, to close friends, to people you are neutral towards, to people you dislike … and then you gradually spread all the positive thoughts you have created to the rest of the world and further. As you can imagine, this was a tough meditation. I didn't particularly want to focus on anyone or anything – especially not myself.

Anyway, I had started on my journey.

Day 2

The honeymoon period was definitely over. I had absolutely no desire to get out of bed. I decided to treat myself this morning and give myself an extra fifteen minutes in bed. However, at 5.05 a.m. my wife whispered to me and asked whether I was getting up. I couldn't fail, and I had to beat my latest setback.

For this reason, and this reason only, I rather laboriously crawled out of bed, put my comfortable jogging bottoms on, and steadily crept downstairs. I made my way into my DIY meditation room and I decided that I needed a boost. For this reason, I reached for a half-used incense stick that was called the lotus flower.

I remember the very first formal meditation that I did in September 2011. This was the incense that was used, and when I am struggling for motivation I often use the lotus flower incense to give me a boost. I also used it on a five-day solitary retreat of which I have very fond memories.

People often asked me why I started to meditate and, to be honest, I couldn't give them an honest answer. At a surface level, I often told people that it was a good way to improve concentration as well as being relaxing. However, deep down, it was always connected to my relationship with food. In a positive way you could say that the last four years of meditation have actually allowed me to gain some insight, and that meditation has helped me to become more aware of my actions. For the last four days I have eaten three meals a day, and haven't had a choice of what I have been eating.

As you are aware, for sixteen out of my thirty-one years on this planet, I have been a dedicated and rather rigid vegetarian. Drastic times call for drastic measures and, for this reason, if I was given meat I would eat it. I wasn't putting a label on any food, and I was aiming to create no attachment with it. This was going against all my ethical and dietary beliefs. Unfortunately, for my physical, social and mental health, I needed to put all my values and beliefs on hold. I had no choice.

As soon as I sat on the meditation stool I closed my eyes and sat silently for five minutes with the aim of arriving, as well as checking in to reflect on how my mind was feeling. My mind felt preoccupied and quite heavy. For this reason I knew that it was going to be a long forty minutes.

It should be noted that not all meditations are both pleasant and happy experiences. I was often reassured by meditation teachers that some of the best sits are those which are difficult both physically and emotionally because you tend to learn quite a lot about yourself. However, it is equally important to embrace positive emotion and to even express a smile if one occurs. It is important to enjoy the fruits of your labour, especially when you are making the effort to wake up when you can bet everyone else in your street is fast asleep. This was a difficult meditation where I was reluctant throughout to express any sort of positive affirmation because my mind was focusing on mundane things. The positive thing was that I was recognising this. I was at the start of my four-week-long journey.

After the meditation had finished, I boiled the kettle and made a fine breakfast tea with milk, and made my way up to the first floor and lay down in the spare bedroom. For half an hour I just reflected on nothing in particular – no electronic gadgets – just me and a cup of tea. This was a pleasant experience, apart from the fact that I could not stop thinking about what I was going to have for breakfast. In a positive sense, I was considering how much butter to put on my toast.

The mornings were a little different regarding what I ate as my wife was in bed. She had told me what to eat but I needed to prepare it for myself. I was so tempted to pile butter on my toast, discard my lunch (which had been prepared for later that day) and wait until 7 p.m. to eat. I had previously seen this as a major sense of achievement. The fact that I was aware of this influenced my decision to moderate my butter intake. I took my small portion of salad to work and ate it alone (I will discuss this later).

Day 3

I had been snoring all night and I woke up with a sore throat. Despite this, I jumped out of bed like a spring chicken. My legs were a little achy, so as I was making my way down to the ground floor I decided that I was going to meditate lying down.

Although the traditionalists would insist on something similar to the lotus position, I often feel that when you live a pretty busy life it is important to give a little. Obviously, it is important not to fall asleep, as that would be a wasted sit. Let's just say that you needed to be in the right frame of mind.

I lit a fresh incense stick, lay down with my head on my trusted meditation cushion, and brought my feet towards my buttocks to create a little stability and posture. I closed my eyes and instantly started to pay attention to the breath ... Good times.

I have a real problem with eating food in public places, and especially with those people who I think might make judgements. Because I am a vegetarian I often get asked about my reasons for being one and, through no fault but my own, I feel naturally challenged. Maybe it would be easier and more relaxed to just simply fit in. Eating at a dinner table with strangers is literally a nightmare for me. I am petrified of breaking into a sweat as this has always been my trademark. When I was young the anxieties started as soon as I felt a little hot. I felt as if everyone was watching me, and especially my forehead. The food on my plate seemed as if it was burning. With each bite I took, my forehead would become sweatier and sweatier. I had one great escape: the beloved toilet. During an evening out it would not be unusual for me to visit the toilet up to three times in the space of an hour. I never actually needed the toilet. It was simply a way of getting away. Apart from in nightclubs, toilets are often a little cooler than the room you find yourself in. I could also use endless amounts of toilet paper to get rid of the sweat. I looked and felt as if I had taken part in a boxing match.

Like I have been doing more recently, I was really good at starving myself throughout the day at that period, often getting to a point where I would become a little dizzy. When it got to dinner time, I would often eat huge portions of things like pizza.

I focused once again on the loving kindness meditation this morning. It flowed quite nicely, and time felt quite distorted. It was a very relaxing meditation with not too much going on.

Day 4

I very quickly get into habits, and it is strange how both the body and the mind adapt to new beginnings so quickly. However, some things are so complex and ingrained that it takes a lot of reflection and contemplation in order to gain true insight. I am very aware of where and how I eat currently. For the last few days I have started to eat lunch. However, because I haven't eaten lunch for so long, I feel very resistant towards eating food in a communal area. For the last few days it's almost as if I have been eating food in secret. I would shut my door and eat my food quietly, and if I heard someone coming I would hide my food. That is so bizarre. I feel embarrassed, but it simply cannot be helped.

I have had a career in eating secretly. I was really big as a young boy and, naturally, people would tease me. Every word stuck and, subconsciously, these feelings of low self-esteem have also stuck. Obviously, I have to take responsibility for this, because it was my actions that resulted in me being very overweight. When I reached my teens I joined a gym, became a vegetarian, and became overly conscious of what I was eating. I was ultra-scared of ever being overweight again. Unfortunately, for the next eleven years or so, my eating habits, my rituals and my obsession with staying thin became the whole focus of my life. Whatever anyone said to me I could never be thin enough. When people told me I was too thin this made me extremely proud of myself and when people jokingly mentioned that I may have put a few pounds on … well, my eating habits would become even more extreme.

This brings me to say that you have to be very careful with the language that you use with people who have an eating disorder. The smallest of things can hit a trigger which could result in the continuation of drastic weight change or, alternatively, a relapse of some sort. An example of this is if someone tells a person with an eating disorder that they look very well. In my eyes this would mean that I had been overeating and that I had let myself go. It's strange how the old mind works.

I had felt a low sense of anxiety over the last few days, and although the loving kindness meditation was having an effect on my positivity towards me and towards others I felt that my meditation needed to be targeted towards concentration and calmness today. I lay down, closed my eyes, and did a full body scan, and became aware of all my body parts and senses.

After a few minutes I started to follow the breath and became aware of whether it was fast or slow, long or short, and, finally, heavy or calm. As you can imagine, it was generally a mixture of both. I used various counting exercises to calm the mind and gradually fine-tuned and focused my attention. I gradually paid attention to the tip of my nose to create a sense of delicacy towards the breath. There is something so natural, so flowing and something so intangible about the breath. It is beautiful, and it shouldn't be taken for granted.

Day 5

I have made it through the first week. Despite this, I jumped out of bed like a spring chicken. My legs. This is what I was thinking to myself as I arose from my bed and made my way to my DIY meditation room. For me this was a massive achievement. I often think of original ideas but I often fail to implement them. For one reason or another, I often talk myself out of doing them. My diet has been moderated very well over this week. I've been sticking to eating at mealtimes only and varying the type of meals that I eat.

On a couple of occasions I arrived home from work and instead of going straight for the bread bin, making some toast, spreading a very generous topping of peanut butter and annihilating it in around thirty seconds because I was absolutely starving, I chose to slowly make my way through a banana. As I said before, I had fallen back into the habit of skipping lunch and had been starving myself most days for eleven hours after my two rounds of toast for breakfast.

I have to commute to work which is a journey of around one and a half hours a day. There have been times when I have felt quite dizzy while travelling, and for this reason I have been known to give in and stop at a local shop to grab a well-known glucose drink. It felt like a sense of failure. However, because it wasn't food, I allowed myself this treat. When I was at university, to get myself through what felt like hours of lectures and seminars, I would sometimes get through up to five of these energy drinks a day. Because of the high sugar content and the long period of time without eating, you can imagine what sort of effect it had on my mood. At times I felt quite agitated and tired. I would often spend a lot of time in my room and would decline many social events. Most of the time I would make a last-minute excuse, such as saying I didn't feel well or I was saving money. I had to really prioritise and consider the most important activities that I wanted to do. I would then put all my thoughts and energy into these. They were my hope in a way, the only time that I could truly get away from my constant battle with food. Naturally, while writing this, I can start to feel my forehead becoming quite hot and close to a light sweat. I feel uneasy talking about it.

Starting your day with a practice such as meditation or self-hypnosis gets you off to an incredible beginning to your day. After completing my practice, I often feel a sense of huge elation because I have started the day by giving time to myself and my development as a person. If the day was over straight after, and meditation was the only thing that I had done, I could say that it had been a successful day. Often I would have days where I had achieved nothing, but this certainly hasn't happened over the last week.

I was a proud man this morning as I sat upright on my meditation stool and basked in the glory of what had been a successful start to my four-week challenge. I undertook a concentration and calming meditation this morning where I followed the breath and focused on certain areas of the body to create more self-awareness.

It should be noted that I am aware that I am starting to get into a pattern of eating habits in the way that I am preventing myself from having any sort of luxury foods such as chocolate, crisps, sweets, cake or cheese. I feel guilty when even thinking about the prospect of eating such foods. I know deep down that the above foods are fine in moderation. However, at the moment I don't have any sense of control over moderating my consumption of these types of foods. And I am also weighing myself every day in the evening (sometimes twice). I do this deliberately because this is when I will be at my heaviest. Then once in a blue moon – when I feel a little side-tracked – I can weigh myself in the morning, when I will probably be up to one kilo lighter. Clever thinking … well, that's what I had in my head. This is quite obsessive thinking.

Week 2

Day 6

It's the start of week two. You would have thought that I may have been getting that Monday morning feeling, with a sense of sloth and pure reluctance to rise from my very comfortable bed. It is November. You wake up and it's dark and – you guessed it – you go to sleep when it's dark as well. To my surprise, and I am not too sure why I am calling it a surprise, I am alert and ready to go. I am intentionally attempting not to overanalyse my thoughts too much, while not holding or grasping on them too much either. I am making a concerted effort to appreciate the highs with a sense of contentment as well as recognising my failures as a way of learning from my mistakes. I suppose it's a sense of moderating the mind. This coincides with the approach that I am trying to take with food. I am certainly not trying to block anything out in my meditation and, with regard to my food intake, nothing is out of bounds. Improving my panoramic awareness through meditation will allow me to have space which will give me a chance to make the correct food choices.

Since starting this process I am becoming very aware of how I eat my food and the speed at which I used to devour big meals because I was starving myself throughout the day. Because I am eating regularly I am not overly hungry, and because of this I am starting – and I say this very hesitantly – to make a positive relationship with food. There is still a long way to go ...

I suppose what I am doing is quite a radical approach in trying to resolve – and come to terms with – my eating problems. I am finding great strength through taking control of what I am doing, and on many occasions my intentions haven't been positive. However, what I am trying to do is to realise that I am responsible for my actions. Yes, external forces can influence my decisions and conditions, but I am responsible for addressing my internal habits and conditioned responses.

I was aware that this could easily be a very lonely process – getting out of bed at 5 a.m. every morning to meditate, that is. I can't imagine that too many people in my street or of my socio-economic status are doing this … or maybe they are. Anyway, what I am trying to say is that I think that it is important to practise your values and beliefs with other people. In simple terms, it is good to meditate with other people. When I have built up the courage to go, I have always found group meditation to be an uplifting experience because it makes you realise that although you are responsible for your own path, you need a helping hand from like-minded people. To be honest, it doesn't have to be a meditation group. It may be a close friend or a group of people who share similar ethics to you. Because of my busy lifestyle, I am currently making a concerted effort to attend group meditations because it can certainly lift your practice, as it gives you a sense of urgency and togetherness.

I sat in an upright posture this morning. My back was feeling a little tense so I made my senses aware and, as I did, the slight niggles and pains passed. They were impermanent; they weren't fixed. I paid attention to the breath and made a dedication to focus my meditation on loving kindness to myself, to my friends, to people I didn't particularly like ... and finally I extended the kindness to the rest of the world.

I mentioned earlier that I was becoming more aware of what and how I eat food. I also mentioned earlier that meditation and mindfulness aren't always easy. I certainly found this out today. I have a real sense of anxiety about eating around people. This is nothing new, and this has prevented me from attending so many social gatherings. Deep down, I am a really sociable person who enjoys other people's company. However, my sense of anxiety of eating around people is out of control.

I had been thinking that it had improved, but when I analysed it in more detail I realised that I was actually partaking in damage limitation, because I was preventing myself from facing those situations. They actually are like mini panic attacks. I will be sitting down and attempting to eat my food, then all of a sudden the sense of anxiety will kick in. I feel as if everyone is watching me. I want to get out of the situation and make an excuse to leave. It could be a trip to the trusty bathroom, or I might pretend to take a phone call. By this point my forehead is starting to drip with sweat as my awareness and mind focus only on this. However, on previous occasions I would hold on to these feelings, putting myself down and calling myself a failure. It wasn't the case this time. I recognised what happened with a sense of reflection. I was naturally disappointed, but I wasn't holding on to the negative aspects of the situation.

Day 7

It was a real struggle to get up this morning. I didn't have much motivation at all. I have found that the important thing to do when this happens is to not grasp or hold on to the thought or you will potentially talk yourself into falling asleep. It is a case of training yourself to get out of bed immediately when you wake up.

I sat on the meditation stool and sat there with no immediate focus or attention. Just sitting is the most important and precious aspect of my practice. I give myself time to contemplate and reflect on everyday life. There is something quite profound about this practice that just works. There is an emphasis on just being in that particular moment, and realising that nothing else really matters. There is no goal – and this is actually quite reassuring, as most things that we do or interact with on a daily basis have a goal.

This practice has various names which include zazen, serene reflection meditation and just sitting. It is crucial to have a formal practice, although elements of the aforementioned practices can be practised in everyday life.

After each meditation sit, I have made the effort of devoting time to myself with no mobile phones, no television, nor any external stimuli. It is incredible to be aware of how tempted you are to look at your phone. After meditating I am now in the habit of making a cup of tea and sitting in my spare bedroom while looking out of the window and watching the sunrise. This is a beautiful way to start the day. I don't really focus on anything, I just sit with my cup of tea and watch the world go by. Yes, thoughts pass by, but each time I direct my attention back to this particular moment because that is really all that matters at this particular time.

I am really starting to have a sense of doubt as to how long I can keep my current diet going. Boredom is starting to kick in and, to be honest, I just feel like going into the kitchen and having a binge on chocolate, cheese, and crisps. It's really interesting to notice this, though, and to realise that if you pay attention to the thought, you will soon realise that your desires pass very quickly indeed. On most occasions, when there is a desire to raid the fridge or cupboard, you feel a sense of shame and regret after the binge. By paying attention to the thought and letting it pass, after only a minute or so, you can turn these habitual thoughts into a somewhat more positive emotion.

Day 8

The best meditations are often the ones where there is a little resistance to meditating, whether it is because you do not want to face your problems or because you have no desire to practise. This morning it was the latter. For various reasons I had woken up a couple of times in the night, and when the alarm went off at 5 a.m. I didn't have too much motivation. My body was aching and my knees felt a little sore. I decided to lie down while meditating, as I generally felt quite tired. You have to be really careful not to fall asleep while practising meditation lying down. Unlike in some Zen monasteries, you do not have someone with a stick who is able to prompt you if your posture is slouched or your eyes close.

Although I have been waking up over an hour and a half earlier than usual, I seem to have more energy in the day. Because a lot of my emotions are related to food, my mind can often wander and get caught up with mundane activity when there is an imbalance with respect to what I eat. However, because my food intake is more controlled and balanced, it almost feels that there is a real weight off my shoulders. I know approximately what time I am going to eat a meal, and therefore there is no need to even consider eating in between – unless, of course, if I was starving, and then I would maybe eat a piece of fruit such as a banana.

Before having my latest setback I had got into the habit of snacking quite frequently, and even overindulging in food during my main meals. I wasn't really aware of this and because I often rush my food and wasn't paying any attention to things like the texture and the taste of the food, I would tend to eat my meals very quickly and almost fail to enjoy them. To pay full attention to your food and what you are eating you could try closing your eyes. Obviously, it probably wouldn't be a wise idea to do this when you are eating in a restaurant or if you are on a date with someone, but you could try it if you are eating alone. By closing your eyes while eating you can very easily block out external stimuli. This allows you to solely focus your awareness and concentration on what you eat. You could almost call this a meal meditation. I have found this to be an extremely relaxing process that has allowed me to make a positive relationship with how I eat food.

My meditation was laboured this morning, and my mind was wandering. Considering that I had been asleep – and then lying down to meditate was the first thing I did after getting up – you would have hoped that my mind would have been quite settled. This wasn't the case. On a couple of occasions I had to take a few deep breaths to prevent myself from falling asleep. However, I have to be positive and show gratitude to myself because I completed the meditation practice.

Day 9

Deep contemplation and reflection are crucial if you would like to make sustainable change. A multidisciplinary approach is needed, and I would never proclaim that meditation alone will enable you to make positive change. Depending on the severity of your eating problem/disorder, you may be prescribed medication or you may be referred to a cognitive behavioural therapist. With regard to my situation I am an extremely proud man, especially when it comes to my pride being dented. If I am to make change, I need to take responsibility.

To support me on my journey (along with dedicating a lot of my spare time to learning and practising different meditation techniques) I have also completed courses, and I hold diplomas in alternative therapies including hypnotherapy and neurolinguistic programming. When I reflected upon the reasons why I have chosen to spend such a large amount of time doing this, I realised that there is something inside me that has an urge to make a change – not just for myself but for others too.

With respect to food I have found that it is very easy to immerse yourself in cycles of negativity. This has an effect on your overall attitude and your approach to life. It can become a terrible burden, something that you rely on to give you control. As well as being your biggest friend and treat, it can also become your biggest enemy. This is why the idea and notion of a moderated diet is so important.

Consider your mind and how your thoughts are constantly changing and jumping from one idea and concept to the next. If your mind is not nurtured and supported through meditation, then it has no foundation to support its development. It will be like a tiger that has been let loose. It is like emotions running wild, and eventually it will succumb to high levels of anxiety and low mood. This is what can happen with food too, especially if your weight is not stable. You will constantly live in fear of putting too much weight on, or of losing too much. People will notice your drastic changes and will start to make judgements about you. Well

… that's what will be constantly running through your mind, at least.

It is important to comment on habits at this point too. Through therapy and self-hypnosis, you can very easily change your habits. The idea is to find the root of your problem or worry to bring about positive change. For you to be receptive to change, your mind and body need to be in a specific state. There are many ways to describe this state but, to prevent too much confusion, I will say that you need to be calm and relaxed. By being calm and relaxed, your subconscious mind will be receptive to positive suggestions and affirmation.

However, not just one session on its own will allow you to make long-term changes. It needs to be practised not just as a formal sit, but in elements of your everyday life. An example of this is when I find myself in a potentially anxious situation where I might be judged or find myself out of my comfort zone. During these moments I have found myself being able to become aware of my breath. I don't make any opinions or judgements about the speed or strength of the breath. I just notice it. This allows me to be in touch with that particular moment, and consequently reduces my worry and fear. From this my mind is clearer, and I am able to be more creative as well as improving my overall decision-making.

Day 10

I mentioned habits yesterday, and how they can have a really negative impact on our general outlook on life. In my early teens and twenties, habits almost became like rituals to me, especially when it came to food. Every day, as I may have mentioned, I would only eat two meals a day: two pieces of toast in the morning and a huge meal in the evening – as much as I could possibly manage because I was so hungry. However, if I was absolutely forced into eating lunch this would mean that I would need to miss two days of eating toast in the morning. This was because, in my mind, this was the equivalent of eating lunch, such as a large baguette or a sandwich with a filling.

Or if I was really struggling to function because I had assignments to write or I was working quite hard, I would treat myself to a very long run. I talked about moderation before, and although I had a stable weight and there was routine there wasn't moderation. It was almost like a fixation on being a specific body weight that was far too low. I would constantly be called skinny, and at times I was a very easy target to tease. I wasn't a nasty person at all. I think that people generally found me quite quirky and, dare I say it, unique. I think that at times people found it hard to understand how I was on academic courses, especially as I came across as quite slow and plodding.

My memory was poor, and at times the way that I articulated my thoughts was quite minimal. I remember that while I was writing my dissertation, my tutor questioned whether I was dyslexic because a lot of my written content was paraphrased and jumbled. All these comments were true but it was because I felt tired and dizzy throughout the day because I was living on empty.

Although I somehow made it through my degree, I never reached my true potential. I didn't start to reach it until I was twenty-three, when I was accepted on to a postgraduate course. For the next few years after that I started to reach somewhere near my true potential. As I have mentioned before, there were blips in between. It was the same situation at school and college in respect of underachieving. Yes, I passed – and I was able to study at a higher level – but I didn't gain high marks which frustrated me. People felt that I didn't care, but I promise you that I really did.

I remember revising for my GCSE exams. When I was on study leave I would revise for around four hours a day. That wasn't bad for a sixteen-year-old boy. The problem was that only a minimal amount of information was being retained because my body wasn't getting the nutrients that it needed. Why didn't I just eat? Unfortunately, my subconscious mind had been trained, and this thought process had been deeply ingrained. Deep down I think that it was in fear of putting weight on because I was really overweight as a child and, as you can imagine, I was teased.

I have a competitive nature, and when I put my mind to something there is a strong will to succeed. For some reason I am quite hard on myself if I am unsuccessful. This leads me to this morning's meditation practice, which focused on positive affirmation towards myself and towards others. On a surface level this can seem like a very basic meditation, but it is amazing how it can have such a transformative outlook on your day, and especially how you perceive everyday occurrences.

Friday, all of a sudden, became very positive and I was eager to make the most of the day.

I am halfway through the four-week meditation challenge. I am really proud to say that I have made it so far, and, if for whatever reason I wasn't able to meditate one morning, I wouldn't procrastinate or be harsh on myself. I would simply accept the current conditions.

Weekend reflections

I think that there is often a feeling in the West that the weekend is an excuse to indulge, to really go for it, and to make the most of that precious time that you have away from the stresses of work. I suppose you could describe it as a form of escapism. You think that as long as you are a good boy in the week – by this I mean eating well, not drinking alcohol and getting plenty of sleep – you have an excuse to enjoy your weekend.

This creates imbalance. Yes, you need to enjoy life and you certainly need to treat yourself. I feel the key to this is moderating your treats throughout the week. By doing so, I truly believe that this will prevent you from resorting to binge activity at the weekend. For example, you may say that in the week you prevent yourself from eating treats such as crisps or chocolate. You then get to the weekend and you end up devouring a large piece of chocolate. You may feel that this may not apply to you. If this is the case this is pleasing because you clearly have a sense of self-control. I am currently practising moderation throughout the week, and it is having a positive effect.

I have never drunk a lot of alcohol mainly because I couldn't handle the side effects. I was very much a lightweight. I didn't like the fact that if I had a big night out with my friends the next day would certainly be a write-off. My relationship with alcohol wasn't particularly positive. Because of this I stopped drinking around four years ago. However, since I started the meditation challenge, I have started to practise moderate drinking. There are not too many beers that I like the taste of, but I remember enjoying Belgian beer. Therefore, on a couple of occasions over the last two weeks, I have enjoyed a beer with my food. That's it, just one beer. I am drinking for enjoyment because I like the taste. As opposed to drinking a few beers while watching the TV, this – enjoying a beer with my food – is very much a social activity.

Week 3

Day 11

It's mid-November, and I definitely have the feeling that it could be a long old winter, what with waking up when it's dark and arriving home in similar conditions. I didn't get much sleep last night for lots of reasons, and when my alarm went off at 5 a.m. I readjusted it for 6.15 a.m. However, at the moment when I was about to re-enter the land of Nod, some creativity arrived. Subconsciously, I told myself that if I didn't meditate then, it was likely that my week would get off to a very negative start. For that reason I shot up and switched the lights on.

My body was aching and sitting meditation simply wasn't going to happen, so I removed my covers, corrected my posture and started to follow the breath. I noticed that the structure to my meditation was very disorganised. This reflected my general mood, as I was going through the process of making some important changes.

The night before was Sunday evening. I was sitting on the sofa in a comfortable position watching television, and generally engaging in non-creative activity. I really wanted some chocolate – so much so that I popped downstairs and grabbed a box of chocolate truffles. I wouldn't say that it was a test, but it would certainly be interesting to see how I reacted to such a situation. In the past, in a similar situation, the box of chocolates would be finished and I would feel a ridiculous amount of guilt afterwards – so much so that I would vow not to eat any snacks or any food that would be even slightly bad (in the way I labelled food) for the foreseeable future.

This time was a little different because I had a regular meditation practice which I was able to apply to everyday situations. This made me extremely open to what was in front of me. I didn't give myself any limits. I took each chocolate and ate it mindfully. By this I mean that I ate it with care and a sense of delicacy. Instead of devouring each chocolate I took my time and made myself aware of all my senses. It was delicious chocolate and, to my credit, I decided that three chocolates were more than enough. There was plenty of chocolate left for the future, and this time I didn't feel guilty for eating it as I didn't overindulge.

The key, I think, is to set yourself absolutely no limits in terms of what you can eat. It is essential to have an incredibly varied diet that has no boundaries. Also, if possible (possibly at a more advanced level), it would be ideal not to categorise food into order of preference. By having no preference you soon realise that food is just food and, likewise, meditation is just meditation. What I am saying may sound a little abstract but I hope that you will understand where I am going with this. If your mind is calm, reflective and can express positive emotion, it will give you space to make more decisions that are compassionate towards yourself and others.

Day 12

When you eat I think that it's important to just eat – nothing else. This philosophy should apply to everything that you do in daily life. People often say that it is a great skill to be able to multitask, to be able to do more than one thing at a time. I would like to challenge this ideology. Doing more than one thing at the same time can often lead to a lack of focus. Energy is channelled into different areas, and often nothing is fully achieved with maximum effort. This can lead to people being demotivated. I have certainly experienced this. I suppose you can link this to the idea of food too.

Imagine if a lovely meal has been cooked for you, but at the same time you decide to turn your laptop on and respond to some important emails. At the same time you have the television on in the background and are listening to the latest news and, also at the same time, your partner is having an in-depth conversation with you about their day. Surely all your awareness and energy have been spread out into different directions making it impossible to focus on the well-prepared meal that is in front of you, haven't they?

There needs to be a certain amount of reverence paid to a meal. A mindfulness technique before eating a meal would be to consider how many people have been involved in actually creating your meal. You could consider which countries certain parts of your meal came from. You could also consider how your food has been transported, and how it has been finely cut and packaged. By doing this you become increasingly more mindful, and you start to gain a deep appreciation of the food that is on your plate ... so much so that you feel that you have to enjoy every mouthful while spreading kindness to all those who have been involved in preparing your meal. All my self-centred thoughts surrounding food are starting to become less fixed. They are open to suggestion, and I am truly starting to believe that long-term change is tangible.

My meditation practice was formal this morning, and it focused on the cycle of the breath. It's difficult to understand why I was so motivated to meditate this morning. I was keen to light my favourite lotus flower incense, but my lighter didn't work. This wasn't a big deal, though. I sat in an upright position and spent the next thirty minutes using various techniques to focus on the breath.

After the meditation had finished, I recited a short mantra to affirm a positive emotion for the day. I then went to prepare breakfast. While I was waiting for my toast to grill, I participated in a short walking meditation, after which I started to spread butter on my now-grilled toast. Using the awareness that I had gained from my formal meditation practice, I was able to pay almost fine-tuned attention to the amount of butter that I was spreading on my toast. It was certainly less butter than normal. I then sat down with no external distractions and paid full attention to eating my toast and drinking my coffee.

Day 13

I really appreciate the time I give to myself after meditation. I often feel that this is just as important as the meditation itself. It almost gives you the opportunity to enjoy the fruits of your hard work. After all, imagine going for a forty-minute run at 5 a.m. every morning over a continuous period of four weeks. Physically, you are likely to be quite fatigued.

It is not uncommon to give yourself rest days to help your muscles recover. It's the same as mind training in a way, but this is obviously more physiological. The more you train, the less recovery time you need. I enjoy running but there have often been times when I have simply not felt like putting my shorts and T-shirt on and going out in the cold. This is exactly the same concept as leaving your bed, walking downstairs and sitting on a meditation cushion. Sometimes it simply isn't fun, but it's almost because you have that willpower and stubbornness that you keep going and carrying on.

I can certainly relate this experience to my experience of food. It would be great to play the role of a third person, to imagine that you didn't have to take control or interfere with what you ate, or that you didn't have to make conscious decisions about what you wanted to eat or what you fancied eating. It would be great if things were just as they are and they just occurred.

When you were a child you learnt to ride a bike and to swim. When you take part in these types of activities they are almost automatic. The skill becomes second nature to you, and you don't have to think about doing it. It's part of your mind, and is set in your subconscious. You don't analyse it or speculate about each movement or mishap. You simply carry on. Although I am very much in the embryonic stages, I feel that with continued training and mindfulness, this would be certainly something to aspire to.

Since starting the challenge, I have been aiming to eat three square meals a day while being very strict and having no snacks in between. I must say, though, that I haven't always been successful. There have been times when I have been so hungry that I have eaten a piece of fruit, such as a banana. This, of course, is a sign of positive eating habits but, because I am very much in the early stages of my training, even the smallest snack could lead to a binge. As the weeks have gone by my approach has started to become more open, and I have been approaching the process with more compassion towards myself.

Day 14

I have to admit that I am starting to feel fatigued. I am currently losing one and a half hours sleep in the morning, and I am dedicating that extra time awake to a potentially life-changing activity. I really do have to remind myself of this sometimes, especially when I feel that it isn't having any impact.

This morning, my practice was dedicated to focusing on the breath. With persistence, on a surface level, this can make you calmer and help you make less agitated decisions. This is because it gives you more space to make more creative decisions. However, if there was one incident in the day when you reacted in quite a rash manner, you might question the effectiveness of your practice and the reasons for participating in such a mammoth challenge.

It is important to remember that there is no such thing as the perfect individual. Regardless of how much you practise mindfulness, you are always going to have feelings of fatigue, anger and general anxiety. The key is to pay full awareness to the situation and, where possible, make intuitive decisions which you do not overanalyse. I think that this is the key.

I suppose that this approach can be taken with food intake after all. I have found that in the past when I have made poor decisions about my food choices, it would often result in a complete downward spiral. I may have started my day poorly by eating a large dollop of chocolate spread on my toast. This would result in very negative self-perception, and would encourage me to continue in the same vein. My day would continue in very impulsive eating. It would be as if I was trying to make the most of the day, eating all the foods that I truly desire to eat. I may come across a packet of biscuits. After indulging in a single biscuit, my mind would quickly become out of control. Then I would eat the whole packet very quickly, ensuring that no one would notice what I had done. Obviously, after these events, I would have a huge sense of guilt and low self-worth. I would then starve myself of any sort of treats for the foreseeable future.

The good thing, though, is that I am currently in a much more positive and resilient state of mind.

Last night I treated myself to a piece of chocolate cake which I ate with a delightful cup of tea. It wasn't a particularly large piece of cake, if I had wanted to I could easily have devoured it in about ten seconds, however, through focused meditation, I was very much able to enjoy every bite ... and the small slice was enough. After I had finished it there certainly wasn't much sense of guilt. In fact, I even felt as if I may treat myself with another type of cake the following week.

Day 15

I was shattered this morning and didn't make it to my meditation cushion at 5 a.m. I had an extra hour's sleep as the practice was starting to take its toll. The positive side to this was the fact that it was nearly the weekend and I would be able to have some extra rest. This gave me the motivation to still practise. I was proud of myself and I needed to almost have a sense of reverence of myself. Personal mantras can be very inspirational and uplifting. By no means do you have to lift the roof off and sing as loud as you can, it's simply the idea of repeating useful phrases to aid your practice and, in a sense, channel your practice.

Words are extremely powerful, and when used in the correct way, they can support you in making positive changes in your life. When creating your own mantras they can be quite open phrases, such as affirming kindness and love to yourself, or they can be more channelled. Over the course of this challenge, I am certainly starting to narrow the content of my mantras and to link them very closely to the sense of eating moderately, and with a sense of compassion to myself. The rationale behind the idea of mantras or repeating positive affirmations is dependent upon the mind being receptive and open to change. I think that you certainly have to have a sense of mindfulness to do this.

At the very beginning of this process my mind was absolutely everywhere, which was very much like my diet and food intake. Also, on a more general level, my mind was generally very busy. It almost felt like four years ago before I started to meditate. I suppose this brings me to the future, but it probably isn't a good idea to think about this too much because it will create anxiety. In some ways I have created very good conditions for myself and have given myself a space to meditate. But what will happen when this challenge finishes? Will I very quickly go back to my own ways? Or will this sense of positive direction stay with me?

Well, I suppose it's like anything, really: you need to continue to practise. If you stop exercising you are likely to become unfit and may suffer physically. Then, after a while, this will result in you starting your practice again. This is exactly the same as meditation. Yes, the challenge that I am taking part in is certainly beneficial and will have lasting effects, but I can't just stop. This is where the sense of fear comes from. I think it might be an idea to dedicate a couple of mornings a week at least to formal practice.

Having said this, though, meditation isn't just about formalised practice. Once you have practised formally, it is important to put all the benefits of your meditation into everyday life. You could call this meditation in action. You have to have practised a huge amount of mindfulness to sustain this through the day; you almost have to be able to be in that particular moment at all times. This is certainly something to aspire to.

Week 4

Day 16

I have spent well over fifteen years practising vegetarianism, which equates to half my life. For around eleven of the fifteen years, my reasons for being a vegetarian were due to dietary reasons. I can honestly say that my mind-set was completely fixed, regardless of what people said to me. With no evidence base to justify my decision, I felt that being a vegetarian would result in weight loss, and would ultimately result in preventing me from becoming obese. This was my thought process.

It probably stems back to when I was an overweight child. I remember being around twelve years old and realising that I was very fat. Naturally, this resulted in low self-esteem, and it got to a point where I needed to make a change. Of course people teased me, and when having minor conflicts with people this would result in people calling me names – which I naturally found quite harmful.

I was always very sporty, though. Well, when I say 'sporty' I mean that I loved football and played as much as I could. I often performed well and feel that I was one of the better players but, once again, I was open to abuse about my weight from my fellow players. Anyway, it got to a point where I decided to make a change, and I don't do things half-heartedly. When partaking in hobbies that I feel motivated to do, I really go for it. I have a strong sense of willpower which can turn into stubbornness. For this reason, I stopped eating meat and became a vegetarian. When I started to cut high-fat foods from my diet, I quickly started to lose weight.

As time went on so did the weight loss. It almost became like a competition. My self-esteem was better, and I started to receive more attention from the opposite sex. Times were good. You probably have an idea of what happened next. This almost obsessive behaviour started to get out of hand. I started to cut dairy products out such as cheese, butter and milk. I started to skip meals and I would aim to fit into extra-small T-shirts. I would look in the mirror and feel I was fat. How I perceived myself was the opposite of how I actually looked. Friends and family would tell me how skinny I was and how much weight I had lost. I didn't really want people to make a big deal of it, especially as people used to notice me when I was overweight.

Deep down I probably just wanted to fit in with the crowd, but this hasn't seemed to have happened in my life. I have always been perceived as being quite different, if not a little odd. I certainly wasn't looking for attention as this is not something that I have ever been at all comfortable with. I mentioned before that I find it difficult to eat with people who I am not particularly comfortable with. I also find it difficult to eat with people in confined spaces. I feel trapped. When going to a restaurant, I always tactically sit at the end of the table so I can leave quickly if I need to escape from the situation.

To return to my original point … I was often questioned about my reasons for being a vegetarian when I met new people, and my responses were always very vague. For some reason, I didn't feel very comfortable.

I had a real sense of urgency this morning to wake up, especially as I was commencing my final week. I did a very focused sit with a real sense of motivation. It was a good way to start the week.

Day 17

Motivation is important in everything that you do. For many reasons it is very easy to lose impetus or enthusiasm. I think that this is often why people fail, although maybe 'fail' is too strong a word. A better way of putting it may be to say 'to lose interest or desire'.

I have a lifelong habit of starting things and never finishing them. The number of ideas that constantly go around my head is incredible. This is mentally extremely tiring, and causes a lot of strain on your mind. It wastes a huge amount of energy, and sometimes it almost feels as if there is not enough time to focus on what is actually going on in the present moment. Because your mind and present thoughts are occupied with other things and life events, you are not able to function, and in a way it becomes a real barrier to your work and to your life. It becomes a central part of everything that you do.

On the other hand, if there is a clear motivation and you have a real sense of direction of what you want to achieve, this type of habit can be very positive. For example, a huge amount of energy has been put into the challenge that I am participating in. Yes, it has affected my sleep and my mood at times. My mind and thought processes have been purely focused on meditation and my food intake – but they have been channelled in the right way.

In week one, I felt that my mood and work performance were being affected by the challenge but, now that I am in week four and my practice almost seems subconsciously automatic and second nature, my everyday performances are improving. Subtle changes have certainly occurred, which I am noticing all the time.

To return to the notion of motivation ... In my teens, I didn't have a lot of motivation. People often asked what I wanted to do when I was older. I hated this question, and wanted to avoid it like the plague. It frustrated people, and I was often perceived as lazy or even a little ignorant. I didn't feel that this was the case, though. I just didn't have any sort of direction at all. Like many teenagers, I simply didn't know who I was and who I wanted to be. And a restricted food intake can be a serious barrier to learning, and can affect your performance.

A good memory is a huge asset to have, and having eating problems certainly affects your memory. I remember that people would often question why I was at university and how I had managed to make it on to the course. Although people often liked me and admired my quirkiness, I don't think that they had much confidence in my ability to succeed in life.

When I look back at how I was, I probably would have thought the same. I think that secretly people were probably concerned but didn't really know how to resolve or approach the situation. I would often turn up to lectures seeming as if I was hung-over. I remember having a part-time job at a pub and the regulars would joke about me being stoned or on drugs. This wasn't the case at all. I simply wasn't eating enough food, and therefore I felt extremely tired.

Day 18

I feel extremely inspired, and there is a real sense of positive emotion. I really do feel good about myself. The change you can make is amazing if you put all your energy and effort into it. With directed focus and concentration, you can do anything you want.

I have transformed the way that I approach food and especially what I eat. I was a vegetarian, and now I eat meat and fish in moderation. And I would also go through periods of starvation and binge eating. Yes, I still feel anxious about eating in front of people. And I feel nervous about eating in public places such as pubs and restaurants. This is something that needs more contemplation and reflection.

With regard to my meditation, there is a sense of calmness and focus. Now that I have built the foundations, it is time to gain real insight through deep reflection. This will eventually result in profound change, which will give me a real sense of acceptance. I am excited about the future, and there feels like a real sense of purpose. Naturally, I am questioning my ability to stick to the changes that I have made.

There is quite a bit of research which suggests that eating problems and disorders are a reaction to periods of stress. People's responses to stress are very different and they react in different ways. Some people get angry, some people like to talk about their problems in detail and others resort to drink and drugs. In the past my comfort was food, and this is probably why my association with food has led to me having quite a negative relationship with it.

People may not believe me, but deep down I am a perfectionist. If I believe in something, I give 100 per cent. However, if things don't go to plan, I can be very quick to give up and lose interest at times. My reaction to this can be quite negative, and I get a feeling of low self-worth. I feel that I am not good enough and that I am a failure. What will happen if my new approach to food has a relapse? I often think, "Do I give up and go back to my old ways?"

I suppose the fact that I am even questioning this is positive as I have a real sense of awareness. I am mindful and paying attention to my thoughts and feelings. This is where this idea of acceptance comes into play. I think I have to accept that there will be times when I eat certain foods that may not actually be 'good' for me. And I also need to accept that there is no such thing as the perfect diet. There just isn't. There is no magic formula to ultimate happiness in life, either. You read about all these incredible people who manage to live until they are a hundred and then people quite rightly ask what their secret to longevity is. Quite incredibly, all their responses are completely different and not particularly healthy. This, then, raises the question: is our life outcome predetermined, or are a lot of our outcomes down to genetics? Well, I suppose that is a debate for you to have. I believe that longevity is down to people's positive outlook on life and, through meditation and mindfulness techniques such as self-hypnosis, you can certainly improve your outlook. Even if you are only committing to, say, twenty minutes per day of formal practice, this can make a difference.

Day 19

I would never proclaim to be a specialist in nutrition or diet. My therapeutic qualifications are in hypnotherapy. My approach is purely associated with the power of the mind, and how working closely with it can result in positive change. You can gain as many qualifications as you want, but this is secondary. Life experience is the most valuable asset to have when supporting and helping people.

I am moving towards the end of the meditation challenge, and it feels as if I am basking in the glory of my success. Tomorrow is my last day. It's an incredible feeling to know that I will have completed such a mammoth task. I have told a few people and they think that I am crazy. However, they don't really know or understand my reasons for doing something so drastic.

I want to talk a little bit about materialism and how this can have an impact on your outlook. There is so much propaganda in the world from people who tell you how you should lead your life. At the end of the day you should be in charge of your destiny, and you should be able to choose the way you want to live, especially when you are younger, though you can easily be manipulated by the media.

I was certainly influenced by the media. When I knew that it was unlikely that I was going to make it as a professional footballer at around thirteen, my passion quickly moved towards music, and this continued to be my passion until I was well into my twenties. When I get a chance to play the drums or strum a guitar it always feels great. I would call it a form of positive escapism. My instrument was the drums. After a few lessons at school, and once I was able to play a few beats, I started to play in bands. I immersed myself in the lifestyle of a musician, wearing the clothes and following the lives of famous rock stars.

I said before that when I get into something, it can be quite obsessive. I quickly clocked that image was important for successful rock stars, and at the time skinny jeans were in fashion. Nowadays, skinny jeans are accessible, and you can easily buy them from popular outlets. In the early 2000s it wasn't as easy. So that was it. I aimed to fit into my mum's jeans. I almost feel embarrassed talking about it now but that's life, and it happened. When I bought music magazines I saw famous people in skinny jeans and they were extremely thin. I wanted to be like them and I would do anything to be so. This naturally led to extreme dieting.

I remember one day when my housemates at university were away. I had the house to myself, and I was going through a phase of paying real attention to the food that I was eating. At the time I felt as if I had put on quite a lot of weight on. Quite ridiculously, I remember only eating a few slices of pineapple during the whole day. Why was this? It was because I needed to be a certain weight to be spotted and to become successful in the music industry. Getting a record deal wasn't just about making music that people wanted to listen to. It was also about having the right image which would allow you to make more money (as well as your record company).

This culture is still rife today, and extreme diets are still advocated in today's society by many national magazines. It is often celebrated when someone loses a large amount of weight over a short period of time. The truth is, though, that no long-term change has occurred here, and this will eventually result in a relapse because the relationship with food hasn't resulted in positive change. The idea of moderation isn't considered.

Day 20

It's the final meditation today. I spent the meditation mainly focusing on the breath. I personalised a mantra to create positive intention for the future. I made a commitment to living a healthy life while moderating my food intake. I also paid reverence to myself, as completing such a challenge has been a huge achievement.

There have certainly been times when I have questioned the relevance of meditating or waking up so early. This process has taught me many things, with one of those being resilience. This has been key in carrying on. In all honesty, though, I have found that I have been happy to wake up the majority of the time and have found a lot of peace through reflecting with a cup of tea after my formal sitting. It has given me the time and the space to prepare myself for the day ahead.

Along with the mantras mentioned before, I also made a commitment to meditate on a more regular basis. I had gone through a period when my meditation didn't have much direction and my commitment was lacking. It was time to get back on track.

It certainly doesn't mean that now I have completed the four-week process that I am cured and don't have to put any more effort in. As I have previously said, anyone can make change – and this includes for the better or for the worse. With this in mind, it can be very easy to reverse all the hard work that has been put in.

Along with formal sits, I plan to focus my efforts on putting meditation into action in everyday experiences. I feel that the key to moderating decisions related to food intake is to find that space where you are about to decide exactly what you are going to eat. To even be in that space will give you a sense of mindfulness. Without that sense of space you are more likely to make irrational decisions. Being in a position where you are able to make positive choices will result in a healthy lifestyle.

As I said earlier, perfection is not possible and we must accept this. Whether you eat a few too many packets of crisps or a big piece of chocolate, the important thing is to notice before you spiral out of control so that you can quickly jump back on track. And also, when you make a poor decision related to food, it is important not to dwell on this too much as this will result in you beating yourself up about the whole ordeal. This defeats the objective of meditation in practice.

The key is not to treat poor decisions with a sense that you have committed a sin. You need to turn this around. With plenty of practice you will actually realise that negative emotion is not related to a particular food. When you go even deeper you may even get to a point where there are no such things as good or bad thoughts. I do not want to go into too much profound detail, but you could regard food as food. You will also realise that when you accept all food types and you eat in moderation, you are able to eat anything that you want. You will have a sense of control over what you eat.

The Three Principles

I would find it difficult to publish this book without at least giving a mention to the Three Principles. My discovery of the Three Principles has only been very recent. In fact, I was only introduced to them while writing this book. Like most other life-changing moments, I find it difficult to pinpoint how they have had an influence on my outlook on life. I think the pure simplicity, yet the profound effects of the Three Principles, were like a light bulb moment for me. It's like that moment when you actually think to yourself, "Oh, yeah, why didn't I think of that?"

The founder of the Three Principles was a man called Sydney Banks. From what I can gather, Sydney was an extremely down-to-earth person who finished his education at a young age. He was not particularly well-read. On the other hand, he was an author who wrote a collection of extremely inspiring books.

Sydney was very clear when it came to his thoughts on wisdom and insight. He insisted that change can be sudden, and comes from direct insight experience. This can be found through having an understanding of direct experience. From what I can understand, Sydney Banks's own realisation of the Three Principles was very sudden. It could be described as sudden enlightenment. He found that every single one of us is just one thought away from change. You don't need years and years of searching, and there needn't be an association with time. With the knowledge of the Three Principles, it can come instantly in some profound way or another. In fact, you may not even realise it.

So here they are ... the Three Principles:

1. Mind.
2. Consciousness.
3. Thought.

The above are three spiritual gifts that give us the tools to create our own world. And, if you want to be a little creative, your life is almost like a film. You are the director, and you truly are in charge of your own destiny. Everyone in this world – regardless of who you are – is on an equal playing field in that all our psychological functioning is made up of mind, consciousness and thought. Thoughts have a direct influence on our mind and consciousness, so our thoughts are really what we need to understand and be aware of.

Now, read carefully ... You can actually have a direct influence on your thoughts. This is because you create your own thoughts. And, even more interestingly, all types of feelings – whether they are positive or negative – come from your thoughts. How incredibly powerful is that? So there you have it.

I will reiterate this once again: you have full control over your thoughts. From my current limited understanding, my view is that all life's answers are right there in front of you. There is no need to search and look for them because you already have them. This sounds very obvious but, on a deep level, listening and reading the simplicity of the words of Sydney Banks can completely change your perspective and outlook on life. Actually, 'change' is the wrong word. This is because you already have a true perspective on life and, as I said, we all do. In a way it's simply a case of going back to basics.

So I suppose the idea is that if you are aware and are able to have a choice over the thousands of thoughts that come and go each day, then surely this can only be a positive thing. By being able to do so, this has a knock-on effect on your consciousness and also your mind. You start to become more aware of your actions and, as positive change occurs, you start to become more open and more aware of your being. By doing so your mind becomes universal, and it expands. It is important to realise that the mind is not like a computer. This is the job of the brain. This is where the similarities with a computer stem from. Sydney Banks differentiates between mind and brain, saying that the brain is biological and the mind is spiritual.

So how did I come across the Three Principles? I was working with a hypnotherapist who was giving me some masterclasses on particular areas of my practice, and he recommended that I should go along to a Group talk. I attended a couple of talks and I was impressed by some of the speaker's theories and outlooks on life. We were moving towards Christmas and there was a Group talk advertised. The guest speakers were a married couple, I believe.

Normally, when I attend talks, I find that I go away with unanswered questions and, to be honest, this is normally quite a normal outcome. The couple have had years of training in the Three

Principles, and straight away, as I walked into the room, I felt completely at ease.

As they were about to start their talk I noticed that there were very limited resources: just two people sitting next to each other. They were ready to facilitate the Three Principles. They highlighted that it wasn't necessarily important to listen to the words that they were saying. And they also said that they weren't trying to sell the theories of Sydney Banks. He was simply the person who had named the Three Principles. Both gave insights into the fact that they have experienced changes since learning about the Three Principles.

From a personal perspective I connected with the words of one of the speakers straight away, as they were very open about their history of eating disorders. Both speakers also stated that they had spent years experimenting with different types of therapies but it wasn't until they came across the Three Principles that they started to make substantial changes.

So what about me? Has the facilitation of the Three Principles had an effect on me? I cannot put my finger on it but, as I left I just felt that a huge weight had been removed from my shoulders which had been feeling very heavy. I simply can't explain it, and by referring to the word 'profound' I don't mean to move away from offering an explanation.

I certainly don't feel as if I need to spend the next twenty-odd years searching and looking for enlightenment. For me, the words of Sydney Banks are extremely simple and, as I said, I have been feeling a sense of ease since that talk. My thoughts are moderated, and I feel as if my mind tends to stay in the moment much more often. As I said, I am new to the teachings of Sydney Banks and I very much look forward to learning more about them.

References

1.   Margaret Hough, *Counselling Skills and Theory*, 2014, Hodder Education, fourth edition.

2.   Christopher Freeman, *Overcoming Anorexia Nervosa*, 2012, Hachette UK, reprint.

3.   Sydney Banks, *The Missing Link: Reflections on Philosophy and Spirit*, 1998, Lone Pine.